Chinese Medicine

Can Help You

Beat Cancer

By

Myles Wray

The information contained in this book has been gathered from reliable sources. However, it is intended as a guide only and should not be used as a replacement for consultation with your Western or Chinese Medical doctor. The reader should consult his or her medical professional before attempting any of the suggestions in this book or drawing inferences from it. All matters regarding your health require medical supervision. If you know or suspect that you have a health problem then seek the advice of a trained health professional.

No responsibility for loss, damage or injury acting on or refraining from action as a result of the use and application of the information contained within, can be accepted by the author or publisher. The author and publisher disclaim any and all liability arising directly and indirectly from the use of any information contained within this book.

By reading this publication, the reader agrees to the terms of this disclaimer and further waives any rights or claims he or she may have against the publisher or author.

Contents ...   Page

Section 5 – Essential Lifestyle Advice …

Section 6 – Your Mind Can Help You Heal …

Section 7 – Qi Gong …

Section 8 – Western Medical Treatments ...

Section 9 – Conclusion ...

Introduction

Welcome. If you have bought this book to reduce the likelihood of getting cancer then you will find some great advice on how to avoid this illness and on how to create more general good health in your life. If you have a loved one with cancer then this book will give you many helpful ways you can introduce into their lives to support and heal them.

If you have cancer it is my sincerest hope that these methods will help you to defeat it. That they will help to prevent it from re-occurring and will help you to attain a high standard of good health and all the clarity and happiness that comes with that.

One of the very worst things to hear is you have been diagnosed with cancer. It is a shocking and devastating blow producing fear and bewilderment. This is especially true if you do not understand what it is, what it is now doing in your body and how it grew there.

With a small minority of exceptions it has come not from unexplainable bad luck or from faults in our genes but from our modern world. From the chemicals in foods we have been encouraged to eat; to the unhealthy lifestyles, the media and other influences have encouraged us to follow. While the introduction of chemicals, modern unnatural practices in the food industry and some aspects of technology has created great wealth for some, it has certainly been to the detriment of the health, welfare and happiness of the many.

Very few people realise that cancer was once, not too long ago, a relatively rare disease. In the United States in the 1900s, cancer affected less than 1 in 20 people. By the 1940s it affected 1 in 16. By 1970 it was 1 in 10. Today it affects 1 in every 3 women and is even closer to affecting 1 in 2 men. **It is predicted to rise even further; eventually in the not too distant future people will be in the minority if they don't get cancer in their lifetime.**

From this we can see how ridiculous the concept of blaming cancer on genetic makeup is, if genes were the cause of cancer and it just ran in families then we would still have the same rates as 100 years ago and cancer would have remained a rare illness !

Some others in the cancer industry have tried to have us believe that the cancer epidemic is because people are now living longer. This does not hold any truth either. Increases over the last 20 years are dramatic, with many incidences of certain common cancers escalating by nearly 1% each year; all of this happening while the average lifespan of a human being has barely budged. What's more are the incredible increases seen in children and people under the age of 50. Cancer has now sadly become the leading cause of death by disease in children.

The only good news is, if you can figure out what has made you sick you can start to unravel it. This is where Chinese Medicine comes in. In the book I hope to help you to understand how your body became weak and toxic, allowing mutations in your cells and cancer to grow from there. If you know how it came about, you

can use this information to do the opposite. That is to undo it.

In China, hospitals commonly mix Western and Chinese treatments together to fight the disease. The Chinese are of the mind set to **use everything available to defeat it**. This is the approach that is adopted in this book.

As most likely you will be taking Western treatments, you can feel very safe in the knowledge that nothing in this book will interfere in any negative way with those treatments. This advice should instead, as scientific and empirical evidence from China suggests, enhance Western Medicines' success rate and reduce the often intense and destructive side-effects from their methods.

I will do my best to present this book in a way that is easy to follow and understand. I will give you a comprehensive plan of action on how to live your life in a way that rids disease and weakness. And instead promotes good health, happiness and strength.

These changes are inexpensive and for the most part not difficult to implement. With a bit of effort and a little time they should start to produce good results.

It is my hope that this information will be of great benefit to you. And if you have cancer I wish my strongest wishes for you, that you will be able to defeat it.

Section 1 – East Versus West

Chapter 1

Why You Cannot Leave Your Care Solely

In The Hands Of Western Medicine...

There are many problems with the way cancer is treated in the West. **Cancer treatments are some of the most dangerous and damaging treatments offered by Western Medicine.** So much so, that in repeated questionnaires over the past 20 years, the vast majority of doctors have said time and time again they would refuse treatments like chemotherapy if they were diagnosed with cancer.

Western Medicine uses a highly invasive and destructive method of cut (surgery), poison (chemo), and burn (radiation) to treat tumours.

Although the purpose of these treatments is to kill the cancer, they can often cause the death of the patient before the cancer has been destroyed.

Chemo is so destructive that it can completely wipe out a person's immune system. Without this, a simple cold or mild stomach bug can turn into lethal life-threatening conditions.

Chemo can also weaken organs like the heart, the liver and the kidneys which can lead to them failing.

Long-term, both chemo and radiotherapies can create cellular damage that can actually cause the growth of new extra potent cancers. They can also leave from mild to severe damage to the brain, internal organs and other parts of the body.

This problem is not the fault of Western doctors as their options are limited by a lack of tools they can use to stop this disease, so rather than do nothing and let the cancer win, they are forced to use these harsh methods.

Unfortunately to top all of this off, none of these Western methods actually treats the underlying conditions that create, grow or prolong tumours. They attack only the symptoms of the tumours not the disease itself. Only by removing underlying causes and weaknesses that allow it to thrive, will the cancer be completely destroyed and stopped from re-occurring.

This is just one area where Chinese Medicine can be very helpful. It is commonly used in conjunction with Western treatments in China to strengthen the immune system and to protect the brain and other organs from harmful side-effects.

You will read later in the book how, no matter where you are in the world, you can adapt all these Chinese Medicine principles in with your Western treatments to protect your body and to enhance their effectiveness.

Chapter 2

Don't Wait For Miracle Cures!

At times it is comforting to listen to the news and to hear that the scientists have had a major breakthrough and are just a little bit away from a complete cure for cancer.

Unfortunately, they have been saying this ever since I was born, over 40 years ago. It never comes true. This is done on purpose because it has a strong psychological impact making you think that the Western system is far more advanced and able than it actually is.

It also creates great spin and publicity for the cancer industry; an industry that charged over $125 billion for its treatments in 2014 in the USA. With such money to be made there are unfortunately many sociopathic minds within this industry who would prefer that no cure was ever found. They would lose their jobs, high incomes and future prosperity; their power, influence and "godlike" egos.

If the West was truly serious about dealing with cancer, it would take very different approaches. It would spend most of the money, including that being collected by charities, not on the highly profitable search for cancer cures but on prevention, where it would be most beneficial. Where it could actually help prevent millions of cancers occurring and truly save millions of lives.

Western scientists have now very little doubt that most cancers, through lifestyle and food choices are preventable. Study after study has shown this. But very little is being done by governments or charities to get this across to the public. Instead misinformation is commonly widespread. Everything from the lies that cancer just comes from bad luck or genes, to the industry spin-doctors who promote that their chemicals are safe for you, to the "we are winning the war against cancer" spokespeople who have hidden agendas to push their expensive treatments. **If we are winning then why are cancer rates still increasing? Surely a good effective health system would have wiped out this dreadful disease by now. Its aims surely would be to prevent illness and suffering; and should not be about making money and creating a massive industry from it.**

Cancer drug companies often charge obscene prices for their drugs. They claim it costs them that much to produce them. Even if that were true, how on earth do they then account for and justify the obscene profits of billions they make on them. It simply does not add up.

If they were really genuine in the attempt to save lives, all Western drug companies and scientists would pool all their resources and intelligence together to find solutions as quickly as possible; instead of the secretive searches for the most profitable drugs that they can patent and turn into the equivalent of money printing machines.

So my advice to you, is not to wait for any cures, not to sit back and be misled by the media or any vested interests, but **to do as much as you possibly can do for yourself to save your own life**. The human body has remarkable healing potential, it only needs to be guided by you in the right directions.

In all my years of practice and in my own personal experiences, I've always seen that those who set their minds to a goal and work patiently with commitment will achieve the best results.

Please don't fall for the trap that some miracle treatment or shortcut wonder herb will come along and save you, but instead put as much effort as you can into steadily following the good advice you will receive in later chapters. This I truly believe is your best chance of survival and success.

Chapter 3

What Advantages Will Chinese Medicine Bring

Over Western Treatments?

Chinese Medicine is very different to Western Medicine. For starters **it is thousands of years older and has been safely used and perfected on billions of people all over Asia** over its long existence. It still exists today for only one reason, that is it works and it works exceedingly well. If this were not true it would have been dismissed and replaced by the advent of Western technologically advanced medicines. It has not been, as in practice many people still find it to be more effective than Western methods.

Traditional Eastern ways are based around the spiritual lifestyle, a search for more meaning and balance in life. This philosophy mingles deeply through the roots of Chinese Medicine. Genuine Chinese Medicine is interested only in the greater welfare, health and good of mankind. Its theories and foundations are based on those harmonious principles. All knowledge is freely shared within the system with the intent of creating a better society and world.

Its advice is inexpensive, practical, easy to understand and easy to implement. Sometimes a little bit of patience is required, but it normally does not take too long to see improvements, not just in a condition but also in general health and overall well-being.

In terms of cancer it is treated very differently; unlike the Western way of just treating symptoms, Chinese Medicine will instead also target the underlying causes that allow tumours to grow. Once it has reconfigured the environment inside the human body, the cancer is no longer being fed. This usually leads to its growth slowing down, stopping or regressing.

To fight cancer Chinese Medicine often strengthens the body's own natural immune defences which hunt and kill cancer cells; on the other hand chemotherapy usually does the opposite and has a devastating impact on the immune system. Chinese Medicine can be used during bouts of that intense treatment to protect immunity and bodily organs. Chinese Medicine is also effective at dealing with and helping to prevent other side-effects from chemo and radiotherapies. This can even allow the patient to remain strong enough to endure more chemo if it has not effectively rid all the cancer.

During Western treatments Chinese Medicine generally raises the standard of living and quality of life of a patient, making those treatments much more tolerable.

Finally after surviving, Chinese Medicine will give you many more ways to keep your body and mind, stronger, healthier and happier while living an anti-cancer lifestyle.

Section 2 – Understanding Cancer

Chapter 4

So What Is Cancer?

In a simple definition, cells mutate (for a multitude of different reasons) inside the body and start to grow out of control, generally forming clusters and lumps of diseased cells. This happens either in one localised area or the cancer fragments and starts to grow in more than one part (which is called metastases). Sometimes the cancerous cells form a solid mass, other times they can circulate in large numbers in areas like the bloodstream.

It is now believed in Western science that there are many forms of cancer, at last count researchers believed there may be over 200 different variations of it.

There are two phases to creating cancer... The first is damage to our cells. If our body is strong and everything is running smoothly then our immune and other systems can take these damaged cells away before they become any more of an issue. Scientists believe this is commonplace in our bodies and can happen on a daily basis in relatively healthy people.

The second phase is where the problem starts. Our system becomes overloaded and toxic and unable, in a sense, to take out all the garbage. From stress or other factors are bodies get jammed up, holding tightly onto rotten cells as they begin to

damage and further take over their surrounding environments. This now becomes what is known as cancer.

Chinese Medicine is not particularly interested in what those cancerous cells are doing at a microscopic level. It does not need to know this to resolve their issues; just as if you have dirt on your hands, you do not need to know its chemical structure in order to wash it away from them.

Chinese Medicine takes a very different view than Western Medicine does. Instead of looking at minute details and trying to see what individual mutated cells are doing, Chinese Medicine always tries to do the opposite. That is it tries to build up a big picture. It's more interested in what constitutional and environmental factors in a persons' life caused the events inside their body to happen, what's keeping them like that and what needs to be done to reverse the problems.

From a Chinese perspective cancer comes from a combination of four factors. They are heat, toxic phlegm, stress and weak energy. It is not always necessary to have all four, but in most cases they will be present. When they are there, they can create a very unhealthy environment inside the human being, which feeds cancer and allows it to thrive.

We will first analyse the effect each factor can have on the body and then in later chapters we'll discuss how to reverse them ...

1) **Toxins And Phlegm** - Toxins, be they natural or chemical, can gather and damage the integrity of cells. They can clog, overheat and weaken the integral structure of a cell leading to malfunctioning in its DNA programming.

Toxins when combined with phlegm (**any sticky goo like impure substance**), can surround and block cells leading to decreases in food and oxygen getting into them; and the removal of waste from them. **Creating a group of cells fermenting, stewing and rotting from both the inside and out.**

To find culprits responsible for toxic phlegm, we don't need to look very far in our daily lives. We are surrounded with unnatural chemicals everywhere we go. And more intrusively we now ingest them in every meal and drink we have.

Many large-scale Western studies have also strongly linked chemicals and gooey fatty substances like sugar and dairy fat to increased risks of cancers.

2) **Heat** - Again like toxins, we can see that heat can be a direct cause of damage to the DNA in our cells. From sunburn to radiation, heat can corrupt healthy cells and start the first phase that could lead to cancer.

It is also a big part of the second phase as heat speeds things up and is seen as growing the cancer more rapidly.

In nature, the heat of spring and summer shoots life forward in abundance, everything sprouting and growing quickly. While in cold winter everything does the opposite - it retreats and slows to a standstill.

The more hot things get the more active they become. If we look at hot steam, the molecules are flying about bouncing off each other. The opposite is true of cold ice where molecules huddle tightly together.

In some Western cancer clinics they test for inflammation (that is heat) in blood samples. They say the more inflammation markers they find, the more aggressive the cancer is growing and the less time the person has left.

So in Chinese Medicine, heat speeds up the growth and deadliness of cancer; but it will also cause destruction in a second way by intensifying toxicity …

In basic Chinese Medicine, if a body builds up too much heat on the inside and there is a presence of fatty or sticky phlegm like substances, then the heat begins to cook them.

It is easy to see this in nature, simply throw out some thick gooey food on a hot humid summer's day. It won't take long before the food begins to dis-colour, stink, rot and putrefy. Insects and bacteria will be crawling all over it. Whereas in winter, if you throw food out into the cold weather, it is like putting it into your fridge. Fermentation and rotting will be reduced to a snail's pace.

Another way to see the effect of overheating is to think of cooking sausages on a frying pan. If the heat is low they will cook steadily. You may get fat bursting from their skins but it will still stay loose as a liquid white fat which is easy to remove from the pan after the sausages have been cooked.

However, now turn the heat up too high and the sausages will burn; their cells will become damaged. The fat that spills from them condenses and turns into a sticky black tar, which can only be removed from your frying pan afterwards with great difficulty.

Heat creates a similar effect in the body, heating body fats and phlegm, making them highly toxic.

3) **Weak Energy** – When our energies become weak our bodies fail to have enough power to keep everything running smoothly and healthily on the inside.
   Our digestion may fail to break our food down fully leading to a build-up of thicker stickier more phlegm like particles in the bloodstream. Our organs and cells may have insufficient power to clean and detox themselves fully, again leading to more unhealthy phlegm gathering and fermenting in our systems.

   To add to this issue, our immune system begins to weaken. This is a massive problem as it is our immune system which creates white cells and natural killer cells to mop up and eliminate viruses, fungi, bacteria, toxins, foreign bodies and mutating cancerous cells. With a weakened immune system are body and our health are left in a very disadvantaged state.

4) **Stress -** It impedes the movement and healthy circulation throughout our bodies. As you tighten up with stress, everything gets trapped and caught up inside of you.

   This helps to increase the other three causative factors relating to cancer...

   Firstly, it locks in toxins and phlegm. As the body seizes and clamps down on them, they get more caught and embedded into you.

   Secondly, the body tries to keep things moving through all this tightness that the stress is causing. So it generates more energy and pushes your circulation more forcefully. This causes it to build up extra heat which stews fluids and phlegm; leading to a soup of toxins.

   It is easy to see the way stress leads to heat; think of how hot and red faced someone gets as they become uptight, frustrated and angry. If they get angry enough then they can even seem to explode into a fiery rage!

   Finally, long-term all the stress can wear you out and drain the life and energy from you; leaving your body weak and your immune system in no fit state to destroy mutating cells.

So the above are the factors that lead to and create the perfect environment for cancer to grow and flourish inside the human being. The body has become completely imbalanced and out of kilter with its healthy natural working state. It has become

overheated, overburdened with sticky toxins and phlegm, over tightened and seized up with stress; and overwhelmed leading to the weakness of organs and the immune and other vital systems.

You may have just one or several of these factors, but more likely you will have them all. Later in the book we will see the many ways to work towards their elimination and hopefully the destruction of the cancer along with them.

Chapter 5

Here Are Some Of The Principles We Will Use To Help Stop, Reverse And Remove The Cancer ...

1) We will look to unblock all pathways inside the body by increasing circulation, and by using bitter detoxing herbs and expectorants, to remove toxic phlegm and other waste.

This will allow cancer cells to be attacked and removed more effectively by the immune and other internal systems. It will also open up the body to allow Western chemotherapy to deliver a more effective result.

2) One of the problems with Western chemotherapy is that while it is trying to cleanse away the mutated cells that currently exist it is failing to stop the addition of new contaminants from corrupting more cells.

This is quite senseless and is akin to bailing out a leaking wooden boat while ignoring a big hole in the bottom of it which is still allowing water to pour in.

We need to both destroy the cancer that is there and at the same time to stop any source of new toxic phlegm and heat from materialising inside the body and encouraging more cancer. To do this we will remove any agitators from the diet and environment. And instead we will introduce foods and other methods that will help to support and keep the internal body parts clean.

3) We will increase the general energy of the body so it can keep itself strong and help to prevent side-effects from Western treatments.

With this it can also begin to do its own internal housework, removing phlegm, toxins and other unwanted substances; replacing them with beneficial high quality nutrients and fuel to power general well-being and a healthy clear mind.

By strengthening the energy, **the immune system will too be powered up to produce many natural killer cells to directly attack and attempt to destroy the cancer.**

4) Through diet and other techniques **we will employ methods to cool the body** internally with the hope of eliminating inflammation and slowing down the growth and spread of the cancer.

5) We will use techniques for the mind to switch it away from stress and instead towards a positive and productive outlook. Eastern Medicine has always used the power of meditation and positive thinking to create health and banish illness from the body. Today, through psychological studies and even the placebo effect, Western science is beginning to understand and realise just how powerful the minds influence is on the health of the body.

As you can see we will be using a multi-pronged approach to increase strength and attack the cancer from every possible angle.

In the next section of the book we will begin to look at some of the tools available in Chinese Medicine to help with our battle.

Section 3 – How Chinese Medicine Can Help

Chapter 6

Some Basics Of Chinese Medicine ...

We have already started to encounter **one of the main theories in Chinese Medicine - that of balance.** We can see how a body that has become unbalanced (too hot, too weak, too toxic and too seized up) can lead to an environment that helps to grow cancer or other illnesses. And how on reversing these imbalances we can regain control and take away everything that was feeding and helping the problems to continue.

Another important fundamental theory of Chinese Medicine is "Qi" (pronounced "chee"). Qi means life energy. It makes perfect sense; every single part of us, just like a plant, an animal, a machine or anything else that exists in the universe, needs energy to accomplish any form of movement or activity.

If our energy becomes weak then we can underperform, can become sick and disease can take hold within us.

In simple terms, you can think of energy in the human body in the same way as you would think of energy in batteries or power from electricity. When we put batteries or electricity into a machine it brings it to life; it animates it. It powers it up to function in whatever way it was intended to.

However, if those batteries start to run out then problems occur. If for example, you have a torch with failing batteries then the light would start to dim. Without sufficient power any machine will falter or not even work at all.

The body is exactly the same, the weaker the energy, the more problems and ill-health it will have. Organs will weaken and be unable to create or move substances or perform their necessary functions. This will of course lead to illness in some form or another. Absolutely everything you do is dependent on energy. You cannot perform a single action without it; every movement and even every thought and emotion depends on it, to bring it to life and make it work correctly.

By simply increasing overall energy in the body you will find that you can cure many problems. Every organ and cell in the body will be more powered up, will work better, be more productive, more healthy, more able to get rid of phlegm and toxins and so forth.

One of the key principles in the fight to defeat cancer will be the maximising of energy in the body. You will discover many ways to accomplish this in later chapters.

Chapter 7

The Two Roads One Can Travel

Within Chinese Medicine...

In a way Chinese Medicine can be divided into 2 separate paths; the first - **the treatments practitioners can give to you will be discussed in this section**. The second - the principles you can follow to help yourself can be found in later sections of the book.

There are many ways Chinese Medical treatments can help and support you in your fight against cancer. In China it is primarily used with Western Medicine in the battle but it is sometimes also just used by itself to defeat cancer. It is a very powerful system.

Although we rarely get to hear about them on this side of the world, tens of thousands of scientific studies and experiments have been conducted in China and other Asian countries showing the safety and efficacy of Chinese Medicines.

In most Chinese hospitals, Chinese Medicine is given an equal position to Western Medicine; solely because it works.

Time and time again, it delivers good results and is well liked and respected by the 1.3 billion people who live in China. It is also very popular in other Asian and Eastern countries, it is estimated that Chinese Medicine now serves 60% of the world's population.

In Chinese hospitals along with medical departments full of the latest Western scientific technologies you will also find departments for preparing herbs, Acupuncture treatments and other Chinese medical modalities. **Chinese doctors freely mix both**

Eastern and Western styles of medicine to produce the best results for their patients.

Treatments can be utilised at all stages of cancer. From boosting general health, strengthening the physical body, empowering willpower and calming the mind; to directly attacking cancerous cells and eliminating the toxic environment which feeds them, to dealing with any side effects produced by the intensity of Western Medical treatments.

The side effects from Western surgery, chemo, radio and other therapies are vast. There are so many ways these treatments can damage the human body. So it is beyond the scope of this book to go into great details of their individual treatments. It is best to consult your Chinese Medical practitioner when any problems arise; they should be able to successfully handle them for you.

However if you follow the advice presented later in this book, then you should find that you can keep yourself strong enough to avoid many of the regular negative issues from those Western treatments.

Now let's take a look at the different forms of Chinese therapies …

Chapter 8

An Introduction To Some Of The Types Of Treatments Available In Chinese Medicine ...

Acupuncture

Acupuncture is the insertion of very fine needles into Acupuncture points which control and manipulate energy pathways and electric fields in the body. Scientists have conducted experiments demonstrating that when needles are inserted into these specific points, electrical activity is increased in these local areas, in Acupuncture pathways connected to them and in areas of the brain.

By manipulating energies many things can be altered.

For example the needles can be used to strengthen the functioning of organs by pulling energy towards and into them.

They can increase activity in parts of the body that have become lazy or blocked up. This extra energy encourages movements to clear the area involved and to fill it with fresh healing oxygen, blood, hormones and nutrients.

Or they could be used to bring energy into the mind to produce a calming and relaxing effect there.

Simply put, needles in the right points can alter energy to create a reaction that causes the physical to change, strengthen and heal.

During cancer, Acupuncture can be used at any stage. It can generally strengthen the body. And can help the mind cope with stress and fear, bringing clarity and peace to it. It is especially good at dealing with any side effects from Western treatments; be it nausea, pain, nerve damage or any other symptoms.

Chinese Herbal Medicine

Contrary to most people's understanding of Chinese medicine, it is in fact Chinese Herbal Medicine and not Acupuncture that is the most widely used part of the Traditional Chinese Medical system. Chinese Herbal Medicine dates back thousands of years, with the first recognised textbook, the Shen Nong Ben Cao, written on it in the first century BC.

As far back as humanity existed in China, Chinese herbalists began to experiment on themselves and their patients. And over the millennia through their direct experience and gathered knowledge of millions of human trials they discovered which herbs were toxic and could not be used, and which others were beneficial in the elimination of illnesses.

They also discovered a multitude of herbs for strengthening and prolonging the life of the human body and mind.

Thousands of text books have now been written, describing in vast detail the properties of each individual medicinal herb. Books have now detailed over 13,000 different herbs, with over tens of thousands of herbal medical recipes describing the treatment of different ailments.

Unlike Western Medicines, each herbal formula created by a professional herbalist will contain specific herbs tailored to treat not just the symptoms that the patient suffers from, but the underlying weaknesses that allowed the conditions to materialise

in the first place. Thus when a patient has been cured from an illness, there is far less likelihood of that condition or a similar one returning.

Because each formula is designed specifically around the status and constitution of each unique patient, a good properly qualified herbalist will ensure that there are no negative side effects; thus making the use of Chinese herbal formulas incredibly safe.

A word of caution, herbs are very safe when administered by a skilled practitioner but are not suitable for self-medication. They can produce strong effects and if used incorrectly can worsen conditions. So please take them under the advice of someone well qualified who understands how to prepare and prescribe them in the safest and most effective manner.

During cancer, Chinese Herbal Medicine **is the strongest asset** you can use. At every single step it will produce good effects. It can keep you in a much stronger healthier position. It can be used to boost immunity; and to attack and change the underlying conditions that allow cancer to thrive.

It is also the most economical and least expensive of all Chinese Medical treatments.

In regards to accompanying Western treatments, after surgery herbs can help you recover and regain strength quickly.

They are very important as a companion to chemotherapy; they will help to boost your immune system and the quality of your blood during this time. This will help to prevent your immune system from failing and help to protect you from getting colds and bugs, which may become life threatening without the bodies working defensive systems. They should also keep you strong enough to prevent many of the other chemo side effects from occurring. They should even allow you to remain stronger to continue longer with a series of chemo treatments if the chemo has not effectively destroyed the required cancerous cells.

Finally, herbs will help to protect the healthy cells and organs in your body from damaging effects that may be caused by radiotherapy and again lessen side effects from it.

Medical Qi Gong

Qi Gong is a set of gentle moving exercises, combined with breathing techniques and meditation. Its main purpose is to regulate and enhance the vital Qi energy in the human body.

It is estimated that over 160 million people practice Qi Gong daily in China. **It is so popular there as it is believed by the Chinese to be the ultimate method of increasing good physical, emotional, mental and spiritual well-being; and longevity.**

From my own personal experience of Qi Gong I happen to agree with them. I have yet to find any superior method of increasing one's health. However, although Qi Gong is easy to perform and learn, it takes time and devotion to produce significant results. It is only after many years of practice that one gains great benefits.

Qi Gong is incredibly important in helping to defeat cancer. It will be discussed in far greater detail in a later chapter.

Chinese Cupping Therapy

Chinese Cupping Therapy is used in Chinese Medicine to treat many different types of disorders.

Most commonly it is used to benefit the lungs and to treat the many conditions they may have.

It's also traditionally used to boost a person's overall energy and in particular to enhance their immune system. This makes it very valuable in the treatment of many cancers.

When a patient has cancer, its use should be avoided on any areas where the cancer is located, but it can be safely used in all other places.

There is absolutely no pain involved as long as oil is rubbed onto the skin before the placement of the cups onto the area.

On the days after the treatment, you will most likely have round bruise like blemishes in the areas that were cupped. These will be absolutely pain-free and will quickly and completely disappear, usually within a week.

My clients particularly like this treatment as it feels like an unusual but very refreshing and relaxing massage.

During cancer, cupping can be used to increase general energy, keeping you stronger in all sorts of ways. And also it is very good at supporting the immune system.

TuiNa Medical Massage

TuiNa (pronounced twee na) is a form of massage that has been used since ancient times to promote the health of the body and to produce healing from many different types of ailments.

Focus is placed on physically stimulating acupuncture points and pathways on the bodies' surface.

Through the principles used in Chinese Medicine it can be used for internal conditions, but in general it is more commonly used for muscular problems.

During cancer, TuiNa can be used like Acupuncture but is usually more used for physical type problems associated with side effects from chemo or the cancer itself.

Chinese Dietary Therapy

Before pharmaceutical corporations discovered there was great profits to be had in the selling of drugs, doctors in Western Medicine used to rely on foods and herbs to create cures in their patients. The founding father of Western Medicine - Hippocrates even famously stated "**Let food be thy medicine and medicine be thy food**".

As the Chinese see food as a weaker version of herbs, they have always used foods as a way of healing simple (and sometimes more complex) ailments; and of promoting general good health and strength in the body.

However, over thousands of years, their methods of Chinese Dietary Therapy have evolved into a very sophisticated and specialised system. They developed ways of understanding and predicting how every food will react in the body and the implications of such reactions. They have classified foods into categories to detox the body, improve energy, strength, mental power, slow down ageing, beautify the skin, tone the muscles, increase the health of each of the interior organs and so forth.

They have not just examined foods but have also looked at how different ways to cook them changes their properties; how eating them at different times of the day and in different seasons throughout the year makes them behave differently in the human body; and the reasons why one type of food can produce very different reactions in different people.

Although there is much involved in the system, many of its concepts are profound and yet very simple and easy to understand.

Diet is an extremely important part in the battle against cancer, so a whole section of this book will be devoted to it at a later stage.

Moxibustion And Infra-Red Mineral Heat Therapies

Moxibustion is used by Chinese Medical Practitioners to stimulate, circulate and increase energy.

It is often used for conditions that involve principles of cold in Chinese medical theories. Cold is sometimes used to describe areas or systems in the body which have become deficient, underproductive and weakened by a lack of powerful warming energy.

The moxa herb is placed on top of needles and lit, or placed in a special wooden moxa box, or more commonly just held over Acupuncture points in a long cigar shaped stick. From there it pushes a special kind of hot energy into the Acupuncture points to regulate and boost the vital Qi energy in them.

TDP Special Electromagnetic Spectrum Lamps (sometimes nicknamed "Magic Lamps") are often used in Chinese hospitals like the moxa herb to boost the vital energy and stimulate healing power within the patient.

Because the treatments involve heat, they would not be used directly over areas were cancers have been located.

As part of cancer treatments, they can be quite helpful in powering up immune energy to help the body's natural abilities to eliminate cancer cells. They can also keep the patient stronger during harsh chemotherapy sessions and at other times to prevent dangerous infections; particularly during cold weather when the body has a tendency to be more naturally weak.

They can be used to restore health and strength after surgery. And they can fortify the general energy and wellbeing of the body at any time.

—————————————————————

Chinese Medical treatments will have a big effect in helping you in your battle against cancer. However they can be a little expensive in Western countries. If you can afford them, then have as many treatments as you can.

But if you are short of money and finding it difficult to make ends meet then only get treatments when it is necessary, such as when you are going through chemotherapy.

Along with these treatments, it is extremely important to try and do most of the work yourself through the techniques discussed in the later sections of the book. All these are very effective and

free. They are vital to giving you your best chance to beat this disease. They will only cost you your time and effort. The more effort you put in the more you will be rewarded.

Chapter 9

How To Find A Really Good Practitioner

Of Chinese Medicine ...

Firstly start with their qualifications, make sure they come from only legitimate Chinese Medicine colleges.

Unfortunately, practitioners from other fields of therapy are now jumping on the band wagon and are often claiming to be acupuncturists; but they have very little real knowledge of Acupuncture and Chinese Medicine. The therapist may have done as little as three months of study in them as part of the course in whatever other therapy they were learning. This produces a very inferior and illegitimate quality of Acupuncture, which often causes painful and unproductive treatments for the patient. It may even cause long-term damage. **A real Acupuncturist will have studied Acupuncture and Chinese Medicine for a minimum of three years.**

Then check to see if they are part of an official register. There may be several registers in your country; but after a quick search on the internet you should be able to find which ones are the main ones.

Next, don't be swayed by a flashy looking chain of shops. Bigger and fancier is not always better; you may find the people who work in these shops have no vested interest in them and work in an impersonal way. Whereas if you attend a practitioner who has their own name on their business, then they will work harder to get you the best results to ensure they maintain as good reputations as they can.

The really passionate people who love Chinese Medicine also tend to make the best practitioners. A very good reflection of their keen interest is shown if they are qualified in several areas of Chinese Medicine. There are four main branches - Chinese Herbalism, TuiNa Medical Massage, Medical Qi Gong and Acupuncture. So what is often good to look for is someone who has qualified in more than one of these fields of practice.

As cancer is such a serious disease, I would strongly advise to find a practitioner who has had experience in treating it. They will have a far deeper understanding of how to handle it and change treatments as needed if you are going through chemo and radiotherapies.

In your sessions be sure to always ask plenty of questions. If your practitioner can answer them with ease in a sensible and logical way then usually you will have found a good one who understands Chinese Medicine well.

Finally, look to see if they generally rush you or show disinterest in your questions, this is always a sign of a bad doctor in any form of medicine. Doctors are here to help their patients, not to intimidate or look down on them. They should treat you respectfully, satisfy all your queries and give you all the time that you need.

Chapter 10

Using The Principles Of Chinese Medicine

To Heal Yourself

In the previous chapters you have had an introduction to the treatments Chinese Medicine can give to help you in your fight against cancer. Most of the remainder of the book will now concentrate on the many ways you can help yourself.

I cannot stress how important it is for you to do as much of these as you can, it may make the difference between living and dying.

Unfortunately you cannot just rely on Western Medicine; it is not very advanced in its treatment of cancer. A great many people are still dying; others are left with long-term physical and mental problems from the serious side-effects of Western therapies.

So it is of the utmost importance to take as much responsibility for your healing as you can; to make yourself as strong and healthy as you can. This will be your best chance at not just surviving cancer but at thriving and bringing as much health and happiness into your life as possible.

The following methods will without doubt strengthen your body, empower its ability to heal itself and help it rid cancer...

Section 4 – Chinese Dietary Therapy

Chapter 11

What's It All About …

It's one of the great gems of Chinese Medicine. For thousands of years the Chinese have been gathering information on how herbs and foods digest and function inside the human body. Through these observations they formed insightful theories and principles that are clearly correct.

The Chinese view diet as absolutely essential to human health. They also believe that it isn't just responsible for maintaining good health, but in many cases it can be used to successfully treat illnesses and restore proper well-being.

Indeed Hippocrates, the founding father of Western Medicine, once said **"He who does not know food, how can he understand the diseases of man?"**

Unfortunately, this notion is now often ignored in modern Western Medicine, for what I would believe to be financial reasons. If people could treat illnesses successfully through the use of diet, then the Western Medical industry would become less needed and would lose vast profits. So it remains in certain business interests to downplay the effectiveness of foods in maintaining health and in restoring it.

There are also many issues in the food industry and the chemical industry that supports it. There is now far too much money to be made by selling the consumer cheaper, mass produced, artificially flavoured and chemicalized versions of real foods. So much money, that those involved are willing to spend a fortune to advertise their plastic unnatural foods as healthy for you. They will not just embellish the quality of the nutritional value of what they are selling but will often also hide any questionable dangerous qualities associated with the chemicals used in its making. We have often seen independent scientific studies come out claiming a chemical causes cancer, only to have a company that uses or makes those chemicals sponsor and pay for a scientific study which comes out to say the exact opposite.

Our Western system has become very corrupted; where the "truth" is controlled by the amount of money and media influence someone has.

When I look at scientific studies these days, one of the first things I do is to look to see who is paying for them. Are they truly independent studies? Or are the people behind them going to become significantly financially enriched by their outcomes.

You will find many of the foods mentioned in the following chapters have been studied in Western Science and have been shown to have strong cancer fighting properties. Most of the studies have been carried out independently by large medical universities and hospitals. I feel 100% confident in their authenticity; as no-one can gain financially from these studies, they are all natural foods that no-one can patent and profiteer from.

All the foods I have listed in the next chapters, which you should try to incorporate into your diet, are all basic foods which are inexpensive and easily obtainable in Western supermarkets.

To deal with cancer through Chinese Dietary Therapy we will follow these simple aims:

(1) We will eliminate foods that pollute and block up the body; and those that are connected to the promotion and growth of cancer.

And (2) we will increase foods that cleanse the body, promote immune and overall strengths, and kill and remove cancerous cells.

There is a lot of information in the next few chapters, so as you read it, don't worry about trying to memorize it all. Just try and get your mind to understand and take in the basic concepts of what you read. There will be a summary at the end of the food section which will simplify and tie all of its parts together, for you to be able to follow in an easy way.

Chapter 12

Eliminating Chemicals That Create And Feed Cancer

There are two categories of food that it is necessary to remove from your diet - natural pollutants and man-made ones.

These foods may be directly damaging your cells, causing them to mutate or they may be creating an unhealthy environment, wherein cells cannot get fresh oxygen and nutrients successfully

into them or eliminate waste products from them. Instead the cells have become covered in a useless, sticky, overheated, chemicalized, toxic phlegm.

The first category we will deal with is man-made pollutants...

For hundreds of thousands of years our bodies have evolved on a varied diet of natural foods and clean pure water. Now in the last 100 years (a small blip in time on the grand scale of things), all that has drastically changed. Everything we eat and drink has been tampered with in some way. Even organic food is soaked by rain with many environmental chemicals in it.

It would be incredibly difficult now to consume foods without any chemicals at all in them; but we can certainly reduce the amount significantly by the choices we make.

Who knows which chemicals are causing what specific damage? Who knows which (if any) are safe and which are dangerous? But since their introduction to the West (or as we are now witnessing their spread from the West to the East); these chemicals have created a mega rise in cancers and other illnesses. So the only logical conclusion I can come to, is that it is safest to return to as natural food as we can get and eliminate as much chemicals as possible.

There are so many different types of chemicals in our foods; from flavourings to colourings, to sweeteners, to emulsifiers, to preservatives and many others. All these however have all got one thing in common, they are all unnatural compounds that the human body has great difficulty in using its natural internal processes to break down and excrete.

If you had a minor illness and for your general health and well-being, my advice would still be to remove chemicals from your diet. I would suggest that if you are buying packaged foods, always to carefully read the labels and study the ingredients. To buy the food with the least amount of chemicals in it that you can find, the ones that seem to be closer to natural products.

But because cancer is such a serious disease I suggest you aim a little higher and cook your own meals using as many natural simple foods as you can get.

It's not always possible, but when you can you should buy organic produce. It has far less pesticides and other chemicals such as the stimulants used to increase the growth of farm animals. Organics are not covered in artificial preservatives or sprayed with chemicals to artificially change their colours and so on.

If you cannot get organic fruit and vegetables then make sure you thoroughly wash any ordinary fruit and vegetables that you do buy. This will at least remove some of the pesticides and other chemicals. Washing them with warm water will produce more effective cleansing than with cold water and it's easier on your hands too.

When you are making tea, you should quickly douse the teabag or leaves in your cup in boiled water for 20 seconds; then pour away the water. This will help wash the tea and remove any chemical residues and pesticides left on the leaves. This practice is commonly carried out in many parts of Asia.

Drinking water can also be another problem; it can be filled with chlorine, fluoride and lots of other nasty chemicals. So get a good water filter system if you can. I use a gravity fed water filter, but with a little research on the internet you can find whichever one suits you and your family best.

As I said, it will be impossible to eliminate our exposure to every chemical, but every one we do get rid of from our diet will help our bodies to become that bit more clean and less burdened; where cells can be fed properly and work more healthily and effectively. Leaving us with greater energy and increasing our ability to deal with cancerous cells or any other problems.

Chapter 13

Dairy And Animal Proteins

Chinese Medicine has always disliked dairy in any of its forms - milk, cheese, yoghurts and butter. **They see it as one of the top phlegm producing foods in nature**. It is far too hard to digest; which in most peoples' bodies makes it leave these larger undigested particles of phlegm throughout them, in areas like the bloodstream, the tissues, internal organs and the brain.

It gathers often in the lungs which can lead to more common colds (this will be explained in a later chapter); and can even affect concentration and disturb the thought processes of the mind.

As a child and teenager my nose and sinuses were constantly blocked with mucus. I spent many years spraying steroids up my nose on a daily basis. They only managed to half clear my nose, making my breathing a little bit more comfortable. When I was in my early 20s I gave up dairy and stopped using the steroid spray. Within six months my nose and sinus became completely clear and it has stayed clear ever since. I can personally vouch that dairy creates much phlegm in the body!

Why is this so important to someone with cancer? Because it is most likely impeding the ability of your immune and other systems to get to cancer cells and dispose of them.

By producing phlegm it will block your body's pathways up, allowing dangerous and other particles to accumulate and gather there.

Dairy is truly a sticky substance, composed primarily of a protein called casein (one of the main ingredients used in common wood glue!), lactose (a sticky binding type of sugar), and fat molecules which are four times the size of most other types of fats.

If you remove dairy from your diet you will find that you give your body a much better chance to allow all its internal systems to fight the cancer. You will also find that as your body becomes unblocked you will lose weight (unhealthy fats), have higher energy levels and feel much better.

There is now a tremendous amount of scientific evidence in the West suggesting that the intake of dairy is strongly linked to increased incidences of cancer in human beings.

Animal protein has also been linked in many studies; in particular red meats and processed meats have been highlighted as being most dangerous.

From a Chinese Medical perspective meat is seen as a rich food naturally high in fatty oils, which gives it heating (explained later) and phlegm creating properties. Both beef and lamb fall into this category.

Historically, the Chinese and many other Asians have eaten animal products in only small quantities; from none at all, up to 1 or 2 pieces a week.

In the past more affluent Chinese who lived in cities ate more meat and richer foods. But Chinese physicians noticed, that as the richer people ate these higher intakes their incidences of many illnesses also increased as well. So the Chinese advice to keep you healthy is to limit intake of meats to small amounts and not to have these too often.

In my opinion one reason meat may be linked to higher levels of cancer is because it is hard to digest and therefore like dairy can leave particles which block up areas, allowing inflammation, fermenting, disease and rotting to take place.

Another big issue in terms of cancer, it is to do with their modern chemical content. Cows, chickens and other farm animals have nearly doubled in size compared to their ancestors 100 years ago.

They are fed a multitude of antibiotics, growth hormones and other chemicals in their short unnatural lives. After slaughtering, the meat is often further chemicalized with preservatives and even things like inorganic phosphate salts. These unnatural salts are used to increase levels of fluids in the meat to bulk up their weight and increase their prices. Studies have strongly linked those particular chemicals to the growth of tumours and cancers.

If you would like to read more from a Western scientific viewpoint of just how bad dairy and excess animal proteins are and how they are strongly linked to cancer, then I would recommend reading "The China Study" by the acclaimed American scientist T. Colin Campbell, PHD.

It is not too difficult to cut back on dairy and meat in your diet. I would suggest you avoid the intake of red meat, lamb and all processed, sliced and packaged prepared meats. To replace them with turkey, chicken, lean ham, fish and eggs. Again try to get the best quality organic meats you can. And remember it is not at all essential to have big portions of animal proteins or to even have them every day. It has been proved scientifically that non-animal proteins such as those from nuts, seeds, beans and pulses provide everything that animal proteins can; and at the same time digest more easily and leave less waste behind for the body to clean up.

When I gave up dairy in my 20s there were no good replacements available, so I just did without. Nowadays there are so many good products. You can easily replace milk and yoghurts with rice, hazelnut, soy or coconut alternatives. Butter can be replaced with olive, flaxseed or coconut oils. Cheese is not so easy to replace but I personally like hummus as a good tasty substitute.

Chapter 14

Safe Cooking Methods

It's quite simple, when you cook in any way that burns food and makes crispy blackened parts then this food becomes indigestible. This leads to it clogging your system and damaging cells within it.

Burnt foods have often been linked to cancer in many Western scientific studies.

The safest ways of all to cook are boiling and steaming. However, don't overcook your food. If you boil excessively you will start to lose nutrients out of the food through the steam. And also overcooked food doesn't taste very good !

Frying gently at a lower heat for short periods of time is okay, just make sure you use fresh natural oils such as coconut or extra virgin olive oil. Don't let your oil smoke and don't burn your food or make it crispy or charred.

Avoid deep fat frying or reusing oils, as through prolonged overheating the oil itself will change its chemical structure, releasing cancer causing agents.

It's very difficult to barbecue or grill without burning the food and therefore these methods of cooking should also be avoided.

Burnt meats are of most concern, studies have repeatedly shown that when meat is blackened through cooking they release the most amount of cancer-causing chemicals.

Lung cancers in chefs and cooks have also been linked to inhaling cancer causing particles in fumes from burnt meats and oils while they are being cooked. **So again don't cook at any high heat that produces burnt food or smoking oils.**

Chapter 15

Avoid Cold Food And Drinks

There is a golden rule in Chinese Dietary Therapy which is to always heat your food and drink. This will strengthen your digestion and help your body get more power, nutrients and energy from your food.

To understand this we need to know how the stomach works. When food enters it, heat is created and bitter digestive enzymes are released. These digestive energies can reach burning temperatures. The stomach itself has a mucous protective lining to stop its own cells from burning up. If you have ever experienced heartburn you will have gotten a little taste of how hot it can get in your stomach. Cooking food in your stomach is in some ways just like cooking vegetables in a pot on a cooking stove. The heat helps to soften and break the food down.

This is why Chinese Medicine always says to avoid physically cold food and drinks. As the nature of the stomach is to heat up to break down food, anytime you put anything cold in it you are

going against its nature; and draining away its vital energy and power to perform. Ingesting cold food and drink is the most inefficient way to digest your food.

If you could imagine cooking frozen vegetables in a pot on your cooker in icy cold water; and then for some mad reason just as it starts to boil to add ice cubes in, you can see that in this way the cooker would use up and waste lots of extra electrical energy.

Now compare this to boiling the kettle, getting it to use the energy instead, adding thawed unfrozen vegetables to the pot and then putting the boiled water in on top. This way the cooker will save energy and use the least amount possible in cooking those vegetables.

This is the exact same process inside our bodies; if we put cold food into our stomach and wash it down with icy or cold drinks, it is squandering our precious energy.

The stomach and intestines will then often have to steal energy from the rest of our body to complete the job of digestion, making us feel tired and sleepy after a meal, and weakening our healing abilities.

On top of that the food will not be broken down properly, so we won't get the full amount of energy and nutrients from it.

And to add to this it leaves heavier undigested particles in our systems, which often create phlegm and sludge inside of us.

To stop any of this from happening all we need to do is to always heat our meals and have small hot drinks with them.

Even something like fruit juice should be consumed at room temperature and not freezing cold from the fridge. This is easily accomplished by adding some hot water from the kettle to it. You can even add more if you wish to turn your fruit juices into pleasant tasting fruit teas.

Cooking foods as opposed to eating them raw is better for you, as the heat helps to start softening and breaking down your food. But never overcook or burn your food as this can waste its' nutrients.

Chapter 16

Fats And Oils

Western dietary guidance has now finally started to emphasise the differences between types of fats; this is something Chinese Medicine has known about and done for a very long time.

We have bad fats that raise dangerous cholesterol and block our blood vessels and bodies up. And good ones that can help things move more freely and work more effectively in the body. This category should really be named bad fats and good oils; as this is a much clearer representation of their properties and the effect they have on our bodies.

Bad fats usually come from animal fats such as those found in red meat; and fats which have been processed and chemically altered such as hydrogenated oils, trans-fats and some so-called over processed vegetable oils. Also natural oils that have gone rancid or have been burnt can turn to the bad side too.

Chemicalized man-made fats should be avoided as much as possible. Our bodies are made from nature and we have only natural means available to dissolve and cope with these fats. Quite often our bodies fail to break them down, and instead allow them to accumulate and be the cause of many diseases.

Cell membranes (the cell walls) are made mostly from oil but it has to be the right type; one that allows oxygen and nutrients to pass into the cell and allows waste to pass out with relative ease.

Unfortunately today's processing and food production methods often harm the oil turning it into a type which pollutes and clogs the body. With the consumption of these impure and unnatural oils, the coating around a cell can lose its ability to allow the free flow of the good stuff in and the bad stuff out. This clogs and blocks it up reducing oxygen and nutrients; and instead allowing waste to pile up inside, causing rotting and fermentation. Ultimately, this may lead to cellular damage which is likely to be one of the causes of forming cancerous cells.

Of course from the view of Chinese Medicine you have not just damaged the cells but the entire pathway leading to and from them. The blood and its vessels are filled with a slimy sludge, just as one sees in arteries which have been blocked up with fats in a patient with high cholesterol. The whole system is now overwhelmed by these gooey bad fats and oils.

So it is very important to remove these from our diets and to replace them with good oils...

Good oils do the opposite of bad fats. They help things slide and glide throughout the body. Organs can do their jobs more easily, conserving energy which helps them to live longer.

If you think of a simple car engine, if it has heavy thickened blackened oil, then this sludge can lodge in parts of it and clog them up. It can cause them to over work and wear out, or even break them from a build-up of pressure.

Good clean oil in the engine will do the opposite, all parts of it become lubricated, move more effectively and will last longer.

Bad fats are heavy, greasy and sticky and can easily accumulate in the body. Once they are in there, it is very difficult to remove them. However, good oils remain fluid like and do not gather so easily. The body can successfully clear away any amount of these.

If you were to dip your finger in and out of butter you can see this effect. The bad fats in the butter will form lumps of themselves on your finger. Whereas dip it in and out of good oil and you will be left with only a fine coating. So although they may contain the exact same number of calories your body is far better able to process liquid oil than it is able to process thickened fats.

These good oils can also mildly help in the removal of bad fats and other toxins by helping to soften them; and then smoothly move and glide them through and out of your body.

The best sources of good healthy oils are mainly from plants... Extra virgin olive, flaxseed, coconut, hemp and avocado oils are all really useful in a healthy diet. You can also get good oil from fish (which get them from eating algae); and from eating any type of unprocessed nuts and seeds.

When buying good oils, try to find ones that are organic and that have been cold pressed. These cold pressed oils have been collected and bottled through cooler temperatures and the molecular structures of the oil has been left purer, more natural and compatible with the processes used in the human body.

Chapter 17

Bitter Cleansing Foods

Bitter tasting foods are some of your most important tools in defeating cancer and the environment that supports and feeds it.

When you put something bitter into your mouth, like a slice of lemon, it causes it to tighten up and squeeze. Your tongue will nearly try to push its way out of the back of your mouth. As this is happening you will notice that your mouth waters. The fluid washes away the bitterness and your mouth is left feeling dry.

The cells in your body simply don't like anything that tastes bitter. They close up against it. As they are cramping up, they are squeezing fluid out to push the bitterness away. They are treating it like a poison; just like that old expression - "**a bitter poison**".

What's most important here is that as the cells push out fluids they also push out fats and toxins as well. This gives them a good cleaning.

The action continues the whole way down through the digestive tract, causing cells to push toxins away and eventually out of your body. You will notice that if you eat bitter fruits like plums and berries it often encourages more frequent and looser bowel movements.

Some of the bitter flavour is also absorbed into your bloodstream and circulated around you. Any tissues and organs it reaches will again reject it, they will tighten away from it, pushing fluids against it and releasing toxins at the same time. **The whole of the body can be cleansed by the ingestion of bitter fluids, foods and herbs.**

Another benefit from bitter foods is that because they have helped push sticky, fatty toxins away from the cells and organs, they have made the movement through them much freer. Because of this, the cells and organs use up less energy while doing their jobs. As less energy is used less heat is produced and the body starts to cool down. **Therefore bitter tastes can help in the elimination of inflammation, one of the partners and supporters of growing cancer.**

Even in our kitchens and around our houses we can see the effectiveness of bitter products. You will notice that many washing-up liquids and cleaning products, particularly those ones dealing with fats, grimes and grease, use bitter lemon, lime, orange or grapefruit in their ingredients.

You can try a simple experiment to see the effects of the bitter flavour. If you get a greasy pan and pour water on to it, it won't do much. If you wipe it about you will make a sludge at best. But if you squeeze lemon juice onto it, you will start to see the fats breakup. If you wipe this, the fats will easily start to remove themselves from the pan.

The natural fat buster and detoxifier in your body is bile. It is produced in the liver and gallbladder. Chinese doctors sometimes in the past have used animal bile in treatments. Can you guess what flavour it is? That's right it's bitter. Even here in Europe we have an old expression - **"as bitter as bile"**.

Bitter tastes will help us greatly in preventing and treating cancer. They are extensively used in Chinese Herbal Medicine to purge heat, phlegm and toxins from the body. In the case of cancer they will help to open up and cleanse all the vessels leading to your cells. Allowing cells to become healthy again and allowing the immune and other internally maintenance systems to remove mutated ones.

They will also help chemo work more effectively, by helping it to move through the open passageways in your body to better target and destroy the cancerous cells.

Many bitter flavoured fruits and substances have even shown themselves to cause the death of cancerous cells in Western scientific studies. They are often shown to be capable of causing the death of many cancerous tissues without harming the still healthy cells mixed with them.

However, there are a couple of rules when using the bitter flavour ...

1) **"More is not better"** ... Be careful when you are detoxifying, if for example, you were to try to drink lots of intensely bitter flavoured lemon juice every day to cleanse faster, you

may end up instead creating violent reactions inside yourself. This may lead to your body over tightening, damaging the processes involved in circulation and trapping toxins inside of itself rather than expelling them.

Also as your cells forcibly contract against the extreme bitter lemon flavour, you will end up stripping away the oils, nutrients, vitamins, minerals and energy that is protecting you and keeping you strong.

So it is best to consume extreme bitter tastes like lemon, lime and grapefruit only in small quantities and only a few times a week.

The proper proportions for cleansing are ...

About 6 to 8 cups of green tea daily – it is very mildly bitter tasting and is easily tolerated by the body, so it gently cleanses.

And one or two punnets of sweet/bitter fruits spread over each day; like grapes, berries, kiwis, cherries, plums, passion fruit, pineapple and so on.

Or you can take them as a fruit juice instead, but make sure they are pure and do not have chemicals or sugar added.

2) Be careful combining bitter fruit and juices with nutritious food. In the West, they claim fruit is digested quicker than other foods. What is actually happening is your stomach

just like your mouth and everywhere else, is trying to push away the bitterness as quickly as it can.

This can have the effect of flushing nutritious food, which has been combined with juices away before it has been sufficiently broken down. When this happens you may be unable to fully absorb its nutrients and the food is wasted.

The exception is green tea; although it is bitter it is too mild in its nature to produce intense flushing effects with foods and is therefore fine to combine with them. The other properties green tea has will actually aid in the digestion of the food, so it's good to have some with meals.

Some examples of good bitter tastes are...

White or green teas; and any bitter tasting whole fruits or pure fruit juices like pomegranate, cranberry, red grape, green grape, black grape, blueberry, raspberry, blackberry, blackcurrant, plum, prune, cherry, rhubarb, pineapple, grapefruit, lemon, lime, passionfruit and Kiwi.

We cannot assume anything about a fruit or any other foods' flavour until we have actually tasted it. When a fruit is not ripe it will usually be very bitter. The more it ripens in the sun the sweeter it will become.

For example, grapes will start with very bitter properties, but as they ripen they will develop sweetness with an undercurrent or aftertaste of bitterness. This is recognisable as although you may have tasted sweet initially, your mouth has been left dry after eating them. When you get more than one flavour in food, you must figure out the likely outcome of the combination. Here in this case the sweetness builds energy and helps power up the detoxifying effect in a gentle way. However, if the grapes were left to over ripen then they will eventually lose the bitter effect altogether. So we must always judge the effects of the food on its intensity of its flavour and not just on the family type it belongs to.

When herbs are harvested in China it is essential to taste and then pick them at certain times to ensure they have the right properties to be used in Herbal Medicines. If they are gathered at the wrong time, they will have the wrong flavours and not produce the right reactions in the body.

Chapter 18

Losing Weight To Help Detoxify And Strengthen Circulation

First off, let me clarify we are talking about losing bad unhealthy polluting and clogging phlegm, fats and toxins. Not about losing good energy and nutrients. As we reduce the body's waste we want to at the same time increase levels of good supporting, nourishing, protecting, healing and strengthening nutrients.

Western scientific study after study has shown a strong link between being overweight and increased levels of incidence of

cancer; the more overweight the higher the risk. This plays into the Chinese Medicine concept again of pollution in the body leading to blockages, rotting and cancer.

Before we discuss some of the correct methods of dieting we will discuss bodily fat. There are two placements for fat inside the body. It is either pushed aside or it's spread everywhere, including throughout the vital internal organs. The fat that has been pushed aside, to the outer parts of your body is not so dangerous; it is not getting in the way or doing much damage. However the fat in your blood vessels and organs is the real killer; impeding the free flowing movement of things, leading to build ups that can rupture and cause heart attacks and strokes. It wastes your energy and tires your organs, as they have to work harder pushing and shoving things through all the fat. It can start to overheat, cause inflammation and rot. Damaging cells around it, causing them to lose access to some of their oxygen and nutrients; and eventually maybe pushing them towards mutation.

Surprisingly, appearances can be very deceptive; skinny people can actually be carrying lots of fat in blood vessels and organs. Whereas some larger people, who have gathered fat over years but who are now eating healthily, have excess fat built up on their outsides, but have clear passageways through and around their vessels and organs. These larger people will be much healthier and far less likely, than thin people with fatty deposits in organs, to get strokes, heart disease, diabetes and dementia etc.

When you diet and detoxify with bitter juices, green tea and so on; the first part of the body to be cleaned will be the organs and blood system. These are the parts the body is dependent on. After this, it will attend to the more external areas. Although you may remain fat for quite some time after changing your diet, your organs and more important insides will have cleaned themselves out. Within a couple of months you will feel and be healthier, happier and have far less of a chance of future serious illnesses.

Here are a couple of tips for losing weight...

The first is not to overeat. Try not to over fill your stomach at each meal. This sounds so obvious but has become quite a common habit for most people. So eat consciously and become aware of it. If your stomach is too full at the end of a meal then it cannot churn and mix enzymes effectively leading to decreased ability to fully breakdown foods. This can easily make you fat, tired and sick. An easy way to avoid this is to simply use smaller plates for meals.

The next step is very important, eat early and avoid eating late. You should completely reverse the Western way of having a small breakfast (or even skipping it as some people do), having a medium-sized lunch and finishing with a big dinner. This modern way of eating is completely wrong. It was brought about not to benefit regular people, but to enrich the businesses and corporations, who wanted their employees to work uninterrupted from 9am to 6pm every day.

Asians still eat their meals in the correct way; **big breakfast, medium lunch, and small evening meal.**

Even older generations in the West ate their meals like this. There is an old Western saying, "breakfast like a king, lunch like a prince and dinner like a pauper".

This is very important to do. And is one of the best things to do to lose weight. Even if you ate the same amount of calories as you would normally do but in the reverse order, you should find that you start to lose weight from this alone. Western studies are now proving this theory is right, that this is the proper way of eating.

Logic and common sense also tells you this is the correct way of eating. You need energy from a big meal to keep you going all day long. At night you don't need a big belly full of food to help you to sleep.

We have evolved in this form for over the last hundred thousand plus years. In those times we would rise early at dawn, get up, hunt and gather food and then eat it. In winter, it could get dark as early as 4 pm, so in the past (before electricity) it was not usual for people to eat late at night.

Our digestive systems are designed to be strong and have energy in the early hours of the day. At night they are not needed during sleep, so the body has evolved to remove energy from them and pass it to the other organs which are involved with sleep and will benefit from the extra energy.

It comes down to this. If you eat at night, your digestion has insufficient power to break down the food properly. It will leave partially digested food in your intestines and stomach. Damaging them and blocking and bloating you. This may cause it to pull harmful fats and phlegm into the body; leaving you only partially nourished and also gaining excessive weight. If you want to lose weight and become healthier, have a big breakfast, medium lunch and small meal before 5 pm; and avoid eating after this time.

Obviously, as I have just said, you should avoid eating at night. However some bitter fruit or juices, or green or peppermint teas can be helpful when consumed in the evening. Because they are bitter, the stomach pushes them very quickly through, washing it as they go; leaving it clean, ready and fresh for the next day. They can also cool and settle you down, preparing you for sleep.

Using bitter flavours will of course also be a big help to losing weight...

To keep a clean and well running digestive tract, you should always have green and peppermint teas, after meals and between them. Then add in bitter fruit and juices for extra cleaning and cooling, as and when you think you need them. This is similar to washing your pans, pots and plates after meals. You certainly wouldn't try to re-use dirty pots and plates again; equally so, try to clean up the digestive tract after each meal.

By following the advice given above (and in the other chapters) you should start to lose bad clogging damaging fats from the body and instead replace them with nutritious, energy producing, health creating substances.

A brief recap on methods for losing weight ...

1) **Eat smaller more digestible portions.**
2) **Eat earlier in the day when the digestion is much more powerful.**

3) Use bitter cleansing fat busting foods like green tea and bitter fruits.

4) Reduce your intake of sticky dairy and saturated animal fats like red meat.

5) Reduce processed unnatural chemicalized foods, which the body cannot handle or excrete effectively.

6) We haven't come to this one in the book yet, but it is simply to increase your "Qi" energy. This will power up your digestion and metabolism to better break down and utilise your food. It will also strengthen the body's ability to gather up and push waste out of itself.

A word of warning: If you have cancer, do not try to diet in traditional Western ways. **If you do try starvation and deprivation type diets, you may end up severely weakening your whole body, its immune system and your ability to fight the cancer.**

This could also lead to a disastrous life threatening effect if you are undergoing chemotherapy which will already be weakening your body and immune system. Under these circumstances, a common cold or bug at this time could finish you.

So please lose weight and detox your body only in the safe ways like I have suggested.

Chapter 19

Hot And Cold Creating Foods

When we talk about hot and cold creating foods in Chinese Medicine, we are not talking about the physical temperature of these foods and fluids; but what we are talking about is the reactions they cause in the human body that generates either some form of internal heat or internal cold.

Heat inducing foods...

It is very easy to see heat produced from foods we eat, because simply we quite quickly heat up after eating them. Heat acts rapidly in nature, whereas cold tends to follow a slower trend.

If we were to put our hands near fire, we feel it instantly and pull our hands away. But with cold, we could quite easily keep our hand in a freezer for 10 or more minutes before it becomes painfully cold.

In the body we get the same picture from hot and cold foods. Heating foods tend to heat us immediately. Whereas cooling foods, slowly cools us down over a period of hours, days or even months.

The most common heating foods are coffee, red or black teas, spices, alcohol, chocolate, fats and sugars.

If you took chilled whiskey from the fridge, poured it into a chilled glass filled with ice cubes and then knocked it back, you will still very quickly feel the burning in your throat and the heat spreading across your chest. It's easy to see this heating effect.

These foods warm your body and release and excite the energy within it. They can give you power to strengthen organs, mind and spirit. They speed things up and generally stimulate the body. They are good for uplifting your mood and improving your vitality.

The downside is, they use up your nutrients to do this. Just as petrol poured onto a fire creates a big blast of flames, and quickly burns up the logs in the process.

Hot food increases your energy, and then burns up your stores and reserves of nutrients. Eventually if you really over indulge, it will even start to burn other tissues and hormones, emaciating you and making you age more quickly. It will literally burn you out.

The best way to use these hot activating stimulants is to combine them in small amounts with food.

For example, if you drink coffee by itself it will burn up your nutrients and reserves; giving you a temporary boost but leaving you to crash afterwards. If however you have a small amount of coffee with a meal, then it will boost your digestion helping you to fully breakdown and retrieve all the nutrients from the food. It may burn up some of these in the process but you should be left overall with a net gain in terms of both fresh energy and reserves.

Another nasty thing they can do is to heat and cook phlegm, foods and toxins, causing serious pollution.

Now with cancer we want to avoid inflammation and overheating as much as possible so it is very important not to overtake these heat producing ingredients into the body, however they produce some excellent effects that do offer help in fighting the cancer, so they will be returned to and discussed in more detail in later chapters.

Cold inducing foods...

In our battle against cancer these foods will help to rid inflammation and slow down the growth of cancer and even help to prevent it starting in new places.

We must remember that cold acts much more slowly and far less obviously than heat. If you consume a cooling food now, it will take a few hours, days or even months, before you will start to notice the effect. Because of this the mind usually does not associate the food as being responsible for cooling your system. However, when you become conscious of these foods and know how to look for it, you will see that these cooling foods really are having this effect.

There are two methods we can use to cool the body through foods. We have already encountered one, the bitter flavour. This is particularly useful when phlegm and toxins are present. Bitterness expels and purges; and as it pushes away obstructions from circulation and your organs, you will find that everything is moving more freely and therefore needs less energy to keep it going. As energy slows the heat it produces diminishes and the body cools. In summertime, we are naturally subconsciously drawn to more bitter fruit to cool ourselves down.

The second and main way we cool down our bodies is through heavy dense cooling particles in foods; like heavy proteins and minerals. About 5% of the body is composed of minerals. They help with lots of functions inside the body; one of which is in cooling it down.

In nature, a general rule is that the denser something gets the more cold it feels. When you put your hand on feathers, then wood, then cement, then steel, you will notice that the harder, heavier, denser they are, the cooler they appear to be. Your dense heavy mineral filled bones will be much cooler than the surrounding flesh and blood.

In physics, they would tell you that what is really happening is if something appears to be cold, it is pulling energy from you. When it appears to be hot, it is emitting energy to you.

We can see the effective use of this all around us. In clothes, ultra light materials are used for skiwear. Carpets are used in cold climates to warm floors, and tiles in hot ones to keep them cool. Even houses made of stone are used in hot countries compared to houses made of wood in the colder ones.

When we consume heavy foods, laden with minerals, they are broken down and pulled into our bodies. Vegetables are an excellent source of them, probably the best one. But cooling particles can be found in most types of food, even in water.

When you look at a bottle of water it seems crystal clear, but in fact, as you read the label on the back of the bottle, you will find that it is filled with many minerals. The particles are so small they are not visible to the naked eye. You will notice that if you touch a bottle of water, it always seems cooler than the temperature of the room it is in. Waterbeds get so cold that even in hot places like California, people cannot sleep on them unless they are heated up. If you're overheating on a hot summer's night, then fill a couple of old empty plastic bottles with water and put them in your bed. You will find at night that they will cool it and you down.

When we eat vegetables, water or anything else containing minerals and proteins, these tiny particles get deposited throughout our bodies. They mix amongst our cells. As living things when we move we create hot energy, some of this heat is pulled away into these cooler minerals. This stops our cells from overheating and suffering any damage.

The dense heavy particles don't use up the energy they are pulling away from the living bodily cells, they merely store it. Once the active cells start to lose power and the temperature drops below the energy stored in the mineral, then a mineral will start to feed this stored energy back to the cells until there is an even temperature again.

You can see this working very simply outside the body. If you put your warm hand on a cold steel radiator or other metal object, energy will start to be transferred from you into it. After a few minutes, if you take your hand away, then get someone to touch that area, they will notice it is warm compared to everywhere else on the radiator. Literally the cold metal has soaked up and drained away energy from you into it. It will now feed that energy back into the room until it becomes cool again.

When you consistently eat your vegetables and gather these cooling elements into the body, you will eventually notice your whole system seems to be cooling down. This is usually good and will slow down ageing and preserve your body and cells just like

the way a fridge slows down the deterioration of your food and instead keeps it nice and fresh. There have been multiple studies linking vegetables to the slowing down of ageing and to the extending of life.

This feature is very important to preventing and slowing down the growth of cancer. The coolness will reduce the heat of inflammation and retard the growth of the mutated cells. It will further generally cool down the surrounding areas and help to stop the rotting and fermenting from continuing.

However, be aware that you can have too much vegetable and over cool your body, leading to a lack of energy and power. This may over time produce cold type illnesses.

In the past, in Western society, most people remember seeing many vegetarians who looked tired, drained and lifeless; often with dull, pasty complexions. They simply consumed too many vegetables, which created too much cold in their bodies and slowed all functioning and vitality down. There are many vegetarians in India, China and throughout Asia who get around this over cooling by adding mild hot spices into their foods to create more balanced meals.

Summary of hot and cold inducing foods...

In summary, foods like alcohol, coffee, spices, chocolate, red and black teas cause activity and movement, and will also generate heat.

Foods that are sticky like sugars, honey and fats will warm things up in two ways – **(1)** by releasing stored energy into the body. And

(2) by gluing up and impeding the circulation and activity of organs; causing them to rev up and push harder, thus generating heat as a by-product.

Foods that are bitter tasting, will cool by counteracting stickiness and allowing free movement throughout the body. As organs have to work less they will cool down. Bitter flavours can also flush nutrients that fuel energy which causes less of it to be created in the first place.

The long term method of cooling the body is to eat and retain cooling particles found in minerals and heavy proteins in foods like vegetables, lentils, beans and nuts.

Chapter 20

Salt

Salt's characteristics are to cool (as it is a mineral); and to move, clean, moisten, soften, astringe and preserve.

When we put it in our mouths we notice a couple of things. Firstly it gently tingles and fizzes. It causes molecules to move.

It also attracts and astringes moisture, so you are left with a wet mouth after tasting it. If we were to leave a small pile of salt on a plate in a cold and damp room, when we come back to it the next day, we will find a little pool of salty water. The salt will have drawn moisture from the air into itself. In the body, salt will hold onto fluids passing through it and keep the cells interacting with it in a moist state.

For example, our tears are salty and our sweat is salty too. This stops these areas from drying out. If you didn't have salt, your eyes would not be able to remain lubricated.

Salt is found in many places throughout the body. The brain is kept in a salty liquid. As babies we are formed in a bag of salty fluid.

A type of salty seaweed is sometimes used in Chinese Herbal Medicine to soften lumps and tumours. As salt pulls moisture into it, when it mingles with cells it pulls moisture to itself and ends up also moistening the cells around it. Salt also fizzes and causes movement, this helps to break up masses.

You can imagine the effect if you leave salty water on a dried out grimy pot. After a while, the grime will soften as it absorbs moisture. And the molecules in the grime aided by the movement of the salt will start to break up and disburse. You will then find it very easy to wash the pots clean.

Bleach is a component of salt. And other chemicals from salt are often used in common soaps and detergents. So salty foods and herbs can be used to break and soften unwanted masses in the body.

We can even see salt corroding and rusting the bottoms of cars when it has been used to de-ice roads after snowfalls. Salt does not heat snow up, but it does start to move its molecules, turning it from ice into water.

In the body salt because of its moving action can stimulate energy; but as it is also a heavy mineral, it will cool and not cause you to heat up.

Salt is very important to diet but only in the right quantities. Overuse of salt can over cool the body and cause it to retain too much fluid; particularly affecting the lower body, the kidneys, hips, knees, legs, ankles and feet. It can also with overuse, pull too much fluid into the bloodstream, causing it to expand and increase pressure on blood vessels. This in turn over time may affect and weaken our hearts and kidneys by causing too much pressure and stress on them.

In general if you have a good natural diet, you need to add a little of the right type of salt every day into it. But if you eat lots of processed foods, you will probably find you're actually over consuming salt, as many of these products have too much already added into them during their manufacture.

Salt is particularly dangerous in processed foods, as because it absorbs and astringes, it can act as a strong carrier to bring chemicals into your body.

The best type of salt to get is natural Himalayan Pink Salt. It gets its colour from the many extra minerals to be found in it. It has been sheltered away from environmental pollutants for tens of thousands of years and is one of the cleanest you can buy.

The next healthiest would be sea salt. However after that, with ordinary table salt, it is best to avoid it as this type of low quality salt often has chemicals added into it.

Chapter 21

The Spicy Flavour

It's also commonly referred to as pungent or aromatic flavours and tastes.

It is characterised by having and creating a feeling of movement through the mouth, nasal passageways and body.

If you smell these foods, their strong aromas will feel as if they are shooting up through your head. In the mouth they often cause a tingling, racing, rushing sensation. In the body they do several things. Firstly, as they intermingle with other parts of you and excite and agitate your cells, they can cause movement and activity. This generates energy and heat, just the same as if you were to start exercising and moving a lot you would end up getting hot. Spices therefore generally warm you up.

However there are exceptions, one such is peppermint, which has a mix of moving and cooling properties producing both a fiery and a cool draughty sensation.

Because of all this moving, heating, drying and pushing, spices are useful at dealing with excess dampness and phlegm. They can be used to clear phlegm from the digestion, lungs, nose, sinus and head in particular.

By moving blood and energy, spices help circulation around the body. This is nearly like exercising internally. They can speed up your metabolism. Make foods move more quickly through your intestines. Burn up nutrients, food and fats, dry fluids and help you lose weight. Also by drying fluids from the digestion it can prevent them from being absorbed and causing fluid retention and phlegm in other parts of the body.

They can have a very strong effect on the lungs by not only expectorating fluids from them but by also giving them energy to breath more effectively.

And they can cause your pores to open which can be useful to allow the body to push out toxins and other wastes through sweat.

However, when taken in excess spices can cause major problems. All that heat can burn up your energy, leaving you feeling tired and eventually exhausting you. It can also burn up your blood and nutrients, dry out your skin and hair, and damage all parts of you. If your pores are left open you can lose energy, and fluids from your blood and vital essences as well. The heat from the spices can also expand your blood which can lead to ruptures, easy bleeding, skin rashes and high blood pressure.

The most serious problem they create comes about when heat combines with phlegm and toxins, this deadly mix can make you very toxic on the inside and is therefore to be most avoided.

A general rule for safe consumption is to be able to taste the spicy flavour, but **if it is causing any sensations of burning it is too strong** and should be avoided.

In terms of cancer the mild spicy herbs like garlic, turmeric, ginger and mustard are very beneficial when used daily in small quantities on your meals.

They will help to create energy and strengthen digestion. Boost immunity by both bringing energy into the immune system and by forcing out wastes, bacteria and viruses from the pores, lungs, sinuses, mouth and body.

Most of all they will activate the blood and move it more forcefully, helping it to push away toxins and phlegm which will help to open up and clear pathways inside the body. There are even Western scientific studies suggesting that these spices can kill and excrete cancerous cells.

Green aromatic herbs, peppermint and peppery vegetables like watercress can also be very helpful in moving circulation and expectorating waste from the body.

Chapter 22

Keep Your Energy Strong

And Empower Your Mind, Body And Spirit

First let us discuss the sweet taste and its properties. The main characteristic of it is its stickiness and its main function is to give us energy.

In nature it is usually formed from the suns effect on plants. The more energy and heat that fruits and sugar cane can get from the sun, the riper and sweeter tasting they will end up being. Because of this, when it is consumed sugar itself can release into the body the stored energy it has taken from the sun.

However there is a second and equally important way that sugar causes energy in our bodies; and that is through friction. Anything that blocks the movement of particles through your body or impedes the action of organs, will cause them to power up and try to force their activity through the obstructions. As they use more energy to push through the stickiness, our bodies start to heat up and rev up our existing energy systems, making us feel more alive and charged up.

When we eat too much sweet food we get a sugar rush. And while this high lasts we will feel pretty good. However, the problem is that it is now using up our existing energy supplies and leaving a sticky, gooey, nasty mess inside of us. So if we take too much sweet stuff in, we can expect to receive a sugar high followed by a slump and a low.

Also the sticky mess left behind can cause phlegm and toxins to get trapped and rot and decay amongst our cells, tissues and organs. This can obviously lead to many unpleasant and dangerous ills.

But sugar in moderation, that is in small amounts of naturally sweet foods (not over processed sugars), can be helpful to the body. It can generally strengthen our energy which will give us a boost in every capacity we have; from digestive power, to immune strength, to increased mental and cognitive abilities. Increased energy simply improves and empowers every single thing in us.

Sweet tastes can feed energy directly into our digestive system, and also its' stickiness can slow down the movement of good healthy foods through our digestive tract, allowing it to have more time to break these foods down and pull all the good nutrients and minerals from them in order to fortify and build our bodies.

In summary, the sweet taste in small amounts can help to build our energy. If over used it can create toxins and lead to a foul sticky sludge gathering inside of us, which will block things up. This can cause heat to build up and can wear out are good energy, making us feel tired.

Examples of sweet foods are raw cane sugar, honey (Manuka is best), dates, liquorice, sun-dried raisins, sweet fruits, pure jams, liquorice and even sweet peas.

Many anti-cancer Western writers have come out strongly against sugar. There is definitely an obvious connection between it and cancer; its stickiness can trap toxins, phlegm and chemicals in the body, leading it to a very unhealthy state of rot and fermentation inside. But this is when the body has gone completely gone out of balance.

If we start to use the methods described in the other chapters to cleanse and detox; then sugar in limited amounts starts to become a very important friend to give us energy and to power up our bodies. And it can even help to energise the systems inside of us which deal with ridding toxins and waste.

We should however stay away from all processed refined sugars and use instead a little brown raw cane sugar or honey etc. as a sweetener to boost our energy when it is required.

Another great source of energy is white rice...

White rice is truly an exceptional food. It is a stable part of meals in Eastern societies. It is a major source (perhaps the best), of good healthy food energy.

In the West people mistakenly throw white rice in with highly processed foods like white bread. They claim that rice too has as equally unhealthy properties as these others. But this is not the case at all. White rice is still basically the same on the inside as brown rice (and just as natural). It has only had minor adjustments, such as the outer fibrous brown husk being removed and the grain being polished to expose the internal whiteness.

The Chinese character for energy "Qi" is made up of symbols for rice and air. Rice simply provides great energy for the entire body, mind and spirit.

In Asian diets some people consume it as much as 4 times a day; as part of breakfast, lunch, dinner and then also even as snacks and sweets. You can mix rice with most meals. You can turn it into healthy porridges and soups. It is a wonderful base food.

Now you are probably wondering why I keep mentioning white rice instead of brown rice; which is generally viewed as healthier in the West. On paper it definitely is healthier. It has more vitamins, minerals and nutrients in it. The problem however is all the fibre that it also contains.

After most people, particularly those with weak digestive systems eat brown rice (or other types of high-fibre foods) they often end up feeling bloated, tired and gassy. This is because the fibre cannot be digested. The body continues to try to break it down but then quite often runs out of energy, leaving the remains to sit in and obstruct your intestines. Once stuck there, the remains ferment and turn turbid, making you feel unwell. On top of that, if you have had vegetables with brown rice, there is no power left to digest them, which means you will be deprived of their nutrients too.

However, with white rice we see a completely different picture. It starts to break down easily, releasing its energy as it does so. This energy helps to power up the intestines and digestion, giving them more ability to digest all the vegetables that accompanied the white rice.

Vegetables have a far greater amount of nutrients than white or brown rice. So anything that aids their complete digestion (in this case the white rice), is very valuable.

Overall the combination of the white rice and vegetables, when put through the process of human digestion, will end up giving your body more energy and nutrients than the combination of brown rice and vegetables would do.

White rice is a very clean food and there is no connection with it causing any form of toxicity or cancer. For hundreds and hundreds of years, generation after generation of Asian peoples have consumed it without any negative health effects whatsoever.

As part of the treatment for cancer, white rice will help keep your body more generally stable and strong, boosting your immune and all other healthy systems.

Finally in this chapter on energy we need to look at stimulants - spices, alcohol, coffee, chocolate, red and black teas ...

All of these produce heat and energy. They are the equivalent of petrol being poured onto a fire - it will produce a strong blast of flames but in the process will burn and use up the logs more quickly.

In the body stimulants will burn up just about anything available to create the energy. This initially gives your body, mind and spirit a boost. However, in essence they are giving you energy at the expense of using up your reserves.

In small amounts, when combined with more cooling, moistening, nutritious and stable foods like rice and vegetables, they can be very useful. They can provide extra power to break down these foods. They will burn some of them up, but will also extract the maximum nutrients from them and make you feel more alive, alert and energised at the same time. So it is always best to only take stimulants when you are combining them with food and never on an empty stomach.

The big thing to remember about stimulants is to use them only in small quantities and only when your energy feels low and you think you really need them.

A little pinch of mild spices on your everyday meals is a good idea to aid digestion; but the stronger stimulants like coffee, dark teas and alcohol should only really be used (again in small quantities) when you are feeling tired and need to be perked up.

As soon as you feel charged up, the key is not to take them again until you start to feel tired and run down. If you feel you already have enough energy then don't go near them. Don't turn them into a daily routine or habit – only take them when you really feel the tiredness inside.

Chapter 23

Other Useful Foods For Fighting Cancer

Mushrooms ...

They have special qualities in Chinese Medicine. They are strongly linked to boosting energy for the immune system. They can regulate and restore health to many parts of the body and are seen as anti-aging.

Reishi (Ling Zhi), Shitake and even common button mushrooms are all helpful.

Western and Eastern studies have confirmed they have some anti-cancer properties.

Nuts and Seeds ...

These are highly nutritious and great for your body and general health. They are particularly good for the production of healing hormones. They can be effective in slowing down ageing and their nutrients can be used in the regeneration of cells.

They are great at reducing cravings and keeping your brain and mood boosted with lots of essential nutrients and energy from the oil within them.

Pumpkin seeds and walnuts are seen in Chinese Medicine as best for helping to make hormones and promoting general well-being.

Flaxseed is also a great all-rounder with a good balance of omega oils in it.

Green and White Teas ...

Green and white teas have similar properties – they both cool and cleanse as they are bitter; and they also activate as they contain small amounts of caffeine in their leaves.

There have been hundreds of studies on the health effects of green tea; most of them suggesting that it has excellent properties for detoxing and cleansing the body. Some studies have even linked it with abilities to destroy cancerous cells.

It generally has a mild bitter taste, so it can be consumed easily and regularly, allowing you to take many cups of it a day. It will cleanse and strengthen the digestive system. And also filter through the rest of the body, gently cleaning it as well.

It is recommended to have a small cup after each meal. You can mix both peppermint and green tea together and drink them from the same cup if you like.

One green tea to be particularly aware of is **Matcha green tea**; wherein green tea leaves are finely ground up into a powder which is mixed into hot water. Thus when you drink it (as you are ingesting the entire tea leaves instead of just flavoured water) Matcha tea will provide you with a much higher dose of both anti-oxidants for detoxing and caffeine for energy. This tea produces a very clean energy which feels more like a calm strength from having a good nights' sleep, rather than the usually over buzzed feeling from too much coffee. It is an all-round very healthy drink.

Beans, Legumes and Pulses...

There are many different types, such as aduki, soy, butter, long, black, broad and kidney beans; and also chickpeas, red and green lentils and so on.

They are great foods filled with proteins, minerals and amino acids. They can be used as building blocks in the maintenance and regeneration of cells in the body. Many beans have as much or nearly the equivalent levels of protein in them as meats do.

You must however, pay extra attention to really chewing beans into a fine paste in your mouth, as they are quite hard to digest. You can also throw a little stimulant like mild spices in with them to aid your digestive system in breaking them down.

Split lentils are particular favourites as they are easy to cook and very high in protein. When mixed in with rice they will form a complete protein. The meal contains all the essential amino acids the body requires. You can also put them with rice and spices into tasty soups, to make a very nourishing meal.

Sea Vegetables...

They have the same anti-inflammatory cooling properties of other vegetables but also the addition of salt cleansing and moving properties.

You can buy many types of seaweeds in Asian stores and even in some main supermarkets; they are commonly used in soups and salads in Eastern countries.

If you prefer, you can buy **kelp or spirulina** supplements and take them that way.

They are a very rich source of minerals and nutrients and have a very cooling nature, so don't take too much at the one time or they can overwhelm your digestion, leaving you tired and weak.

You should mix mild stimulants with them to aid your digestive system in breaking them down.

Peppermint ...

Peppermint is wonderful for the digestion. It is also a good expectorant, can move circulation and can help the immune system.

It is easy to take as peppermint tea. But if you don't like that, then try temporarily taking peppermint sweets until you acquire a liking for its flavour.

It moves, cleans, warms and then cools. Its' taste can feel fiery and then become like a cool breeze.

It helps to create energy in the stomach and intestines. It cleans them, then cools them and leaves them fresh and ready, prepared for the next meal. You can even use it to gurgle with, clean your mouth and freshen up your breath (just like you see it being used in many bottles of mouthwash).

It is great for treating many digestive disorders, particularly those involving gas, bloating and pains. You should have a small cup of it with or after every meal.

Ginger ...

It can be very good at strengthening and settling a weak digestive system.

Mix it with other spices and herbs; and add small quantities of them to your rice and vegetable meals.

Garlic and Turmeric ...

Both of these spices are mild and well tolerated in the body; producing just a minimum of extra heat.

They can be very effective at increasing circulation, which in turn can help discard and expectorate phlegm and destroyed cancerous cells from your body.

They can both boost your immune system and help to guard the body from invading bacteria and viruses. In China, garlic is commonly taken in winter to prevent cold and flu.

Mix a small amount daily on to your rice and vegetables with other herbs and spices.

Cinnamon ...

Cinnamon is a great spice that is not too over-heating.

It is excellent at promoting general and hormonal health in the body.

In Chinese Medicine it is used to regulate and restore health to many parts of the body, but is especially suited to people who feel tired, run down and cold.

Alcohol ...

Alcohol can be made from many different sources. Some of these will give the alcohol extra unique qualities along with its base of heat and activity.

For example, wines made from grapes tend to have heating, bitter and activating qualities.

If you have a clean, phlegm and toxic free body, then these will just heat and dry fluids. But if you do have a poor diet and have gathered phlegm and toxins within, then these will most likely bake and congeal them into smaller more dangerous elements.

You will notice in many Western studies on alcohol that one study suggests it has beneficial properties while another says it is damaging. As you can now understand, it all depends on the type of people you put them into. Generally they are bad for people who are already hot and toxic. And good for those who are cold and deficient in energy.

With cancer you should avoid it until you become cleaner on the inside; then just like coffee and sugar, a little of it can be helpful under the right circumstances - that is when your energy is weak and you need a bit of a boost.

In small quantities, alcohol can increase energy levels, strengthen digestion and immunity, move your circulation and boost the mind and spirit. From this perspective it can be quite useful.

But obviously avoid alcoholic drinks that are over processed and full of sugar and chemicals.

Chapter 24

Summary Of Chinese Dietary Therapy

In The Treatment And Prevention Of Cancer

From what we have learnt so far, we can see that cancer is all about cells and their environments being damaged by heat and pollution.

Cancer appears to have two phases - the initial damage to the integral make-up of the cells; and then the build-up of toxins and pollution around the infrastructure of the cells, which limits their oxygen and nutrients and instead causes them to rot and ferment until they eventually mutate and multiply out of control.

From the chapters on diet we have learnt our foods can play a major role in encouraging or discouraging the formation of cancerous cells and the systems that feed them.

In simple terms, foods that heat, inflame, congest, impede, pollute, putrefy and ferment will encourage cancer and its growth.

Whereas foods that cleanse, detox, expectorate, purge and energise will retard cancers growth and formation.

Based on these ideas I will now present a straightforward general list of toxic foods you should remove from your diet and another list of healing foods that you should consume often. Following both lists will help you significantly in your battle against cancer.

Damaging Foods To Reduce Or Remove From Your Diet...

Dairy – Cow or animal milk, cheese, butter and yoghurts. (Replace them with rice, soy, coconut, almond, hummus or olive oil alternatives).

Meat - Red meats, lamb, bacon, sausages and processed / preserved meats like packaged sliced ham or chicken. (Replace them with organic chicken, turkey, lean ham, fish, eggs, lentils or beans).

Fats - Trans fats, hydrogenated fats and processed vegetable oils. (Replace them with extra virgin olive oil, flaxseed oil, coconut oil or hemp oils).

Junk Foods - Processed packaged foods, unhealthy take-aways, fast foods, sweets, cakes, crisps and so on. Basically any type of man-made chemicalized unnatural foods. (Replace with home cooked meals and snacks from organic and natural ingredients).

Onions and Hot Chilli Style Peppers – The nature of onions is to heat and astringe; this locks in toxins and inflammation, leading to fermenting putrid blockages in the body. They should only be taken if your diet is 100% natural and you have no signs of toxins in your system.

Chilli style peppers are just too hot. They will burn and damage cells. If there are pre-existing toxins and phlegm in the body then these will congeal and thicken with the intense heat, making them even more embedded and dangerous. (Replace these with mild spices that give plenty of flavour but do not burn or heat excessively).

Bananas – They are not necessarily a bad food, there is nothing toxic within them. But they do have properties that are gooey and sticky. All you have to do is to put a banana in your mouth and you will taste the thick sludge that is created.

This is perfect under the right conditions – that is if the body is hot and dry (like in the climates that bananas grow in). In these circumstances they can be used to help create moisture inside of us.

However, as we have seen that cancer is related to phlegm, fats and toxins congesting in the pathways inside the body, then it is best to avoid phlegm producing bananas in your diet. They could add tacky goo to block things up further and interfere with the removal of toxins and cancerous cells from the body.

All of the foods in our list above can generally block you up and clog up your body's network of pathways; leading to inflammation, damage and decay.

Helpful Healing Foods To Add Into Your Diet...

Bitter Fruits and their Pure Juices – Such as pomegranates, black grapes, red grapes, green grapes, plums, passion fruit, rhubarb, prunes, kiwi fruits, cherries, pineapples, blackcurrants, cranberries, raspberries, blueberries and little amounts of lemon, lime and grapefruit.

They will help to cleanse, destroy and purge unwanted substances from the body, leaving it cleaner and cooler.

Take 1 to 2 punnets or glasses of them a day.

Green and White Teas – These are cleansing and cooling, just like bitter fruits, but they act in a weaker way which allows you to take plenty of them.

Have about 4 to 8 cups of them each day.

Vegetables - Any type of them (apart from onions and hot peppers) will over time build up levels of cooling minerals to help rid inflammation in the body. They also support general health in lots of other ways.

They are hard to digest so it is best to serve them with white rice and a little spice (turmeric, garlic, ginger etc.). It's good to have a varied mix of them as this will provide lots of different nutrients.

Sea Vegetables – Such as any of the types of edible seaweeds, like dulse, kelp and spirulina etc. They are a more intensive cooler version of vegetables.

You can put them in soups, salads or just take them as supplements.

They are best taken with stimulants to help them to digest.

Spices – They can stimulate energy, move and increase circulation, and expectorate phlegm and toxins from the body. They are also very good at supporting digestion and the immune system too.

Take them daily in small doses with meals. The best ones are turmeric, garlic, ginger, mustard and the mild tasting ones (stay away from anything that burns your mouth).

In large amounts they can overheat and damage you - so don't take too much of them.

Fragrant Green Herbs and Plants - Like peppermint, parsley and watercress. They have similar properties to spices, but are usually gentler on the body and have cooling properties instead of heating ones.

Peppermint is a particularly helpful one - very useful for easing and stimulating the digestion; good for the immune system and for expectorating phlegm from the lungs and head. It should be taken daily.

Nuts and Seeds – These are filled with cooling minerals, energising oils and lots of other nutrients. They are great for supporting the mind and for nourishing overall health and well-being.

Walnuts and pumpkin seeds are particularly beneficial.

Mushrooms and Cinnamon – Both are good for all-round health. In particular they can boost the immune and cell regenerating hormonal systems.

Cinnamon's nature is to warm, so it works better when the body is cold. You only need a little sprinkle of cinnamon powder when you need to use it. You can put it on food or mix it in with teas.

Mushrooms have been shown to be helpful in treating cancer, they are often given to cancer patients in Japanese hospitals. You should try to have them often.

Salt - Amongst many other good qualities, it helps to cool and to dissolve masses in the body.

Add a little of it to your main daily meal.

Himalayan Pink Salt is the cleanest and healthiest.

White Rice – This is a very important essential clean food to build everyday strength and energy in the body. To keep it regulated and running in good shape.

Have it as your main meal in the day. You can mix it in with your vegetables; and with lentils, beans or small amounts of meats like chicken, lean ham, turkey, fish or eggs.

It will be of great help to keep you stronger and more stable if you do this.

To keep it tasty and interesting you can add different amounts of mild spices like turmeric, garlic, ginger and mustard; green herbs like basil, oregano and parsley; and other flavourings like soy sauce, organic stock cubes, organic tomato ketchup and Himalayan salt.

Stimulants - Use these to perk up your body when you are feeling tired, run down and cold. They are best taken with food and are great at getting things going again, bringing your energy and vitality back and putting you into a positive mind frame.

But (with the exception of mild spices) don't turn stimulants into routine daily habits. Instead listen to your body and only take them as required or else they will start to overheat you, may create extra toxins in your system and also burn up your reserves of nutrients excessively.

Coffee, Chocolate, Red and Black Teas - Their properties are to heat, enliven, energise and purge.

Small amounts with food are helpful to get a weak digestive system going again.

Alcohol – It heats, energises, helps a weak heart, moves circulation and perks up the spirit and mind when it's taken in small quantities.

Raw Cane Sugar – It boosts digestive and general energy in the body. It's very sticky so use it sparingly.

Peppermint Sweets – They are probably the healthiest of all sweets. If you have to have sweets then go for these.

They can be quite helpful to weak or clogged-up digestive systems.

Honey – It can boost general energy and also has mild antiseptic qualities. However, out of all the honeys Manuka Honey is the best as it is obtained by bees from tea tree flowers and this gives it much stronger cleansing properties.

Like all other stimulants it should still only be used when required and in small quantities, just enough to get you energised again.

Liquorice – It's good for a weak digestive system and for boosting general energy levels.

It is best to take it in root form as a tea.

Again only take it when required to perk up your system, and stop taking it when this is achieved or you will risk overheating and creating toxins in your body.

Good Oils - Organic extra virgin olive oil, hemp oil, flaxseed oil, coconut oil and fish oils are all beneficial. They will do many things to boost overall health in the body; including supporting hormonal, organ, joint, heart and brain health. They will help things slide and glide inside of you and will help to get unwanted things to be moved through and ejected from your system.

Extra virgin olive oil is probably the most versatile and best for everyday cooking and for pouring directly onto food.

Use it instead of butter and pour it onto rice, salads, vegetables, potatoes, pasta and meats. If you want to you can mix it with a little salt, spices and green herbs to give it some extra taste. Add about a tablespoon of it on to your food every day.

General Guidelines For Healthy Eating ...

Buy organic foods whenever it is possible - they are the cleanest and purest foods we have left on our planet.

To keep your digestion at its strongest and most effective, have a big breakfast, a medium lunch and a small dinner. After 5pm only drink teas or have bitter fruits or their pure juices.

Don't overfill your stomach, leave room for it to churn and digest your food properly.

Avoid cold foods and drinks. They will weaken your digestive system, create phlegm and deplete your general energy. Heat your foods to start them breaking down (but don't overcook them as it will deplete their nutrients). If you are having a salad or some raw food then have a little spice on it; and also have a hot cup of tea with it to give your digestion extra energy.

Don't eat any burnt food - it is indigestible and is strongly linked to releasing cancer-causing agents in the body.

The bottom line ...

Cancer is all about heat, obstructions and toxins. So the trend of your diet should generally be about detoxifying and cooling. But be careful not to try to force the body too quickly as this will most likely throw it out of balance. Your body needs to cleanse and remove cancerous growths but it still needs to keep every other part of it nourished, energised, supported and healthy.

So your diet must be kept in a realm where you are cleansing but also building and strengthening all your other assets - your physical body and its organs (particularly the immune system); and your mind, emotions and spirit too.

Ideally we want to cleanse, remove the cancer and make you thrive with great health at the same time.

Section 5 – Essential Lifestyle Advice

Chapter 25

The Importance Of Sleep...

Sleep is absolutely crucial for a number of reasons...

1) Western scientific studies have shown that tumours can grow 2 to 3 times faster in animals that are deprived of sleep. Other studies have shown that people who get short amounts of sleep, disturbed sleep or who work night shifts (when the body should be at rest), all had considerably higher risks of developing cancers in comparison to those who get reasonably healthy amounts of sleep.

2) Sleep helps us to regain general balance in our bodies. If we keep running our systems for too long we will simply burn out and crash. Sleeps helps us to prevent this by turning ourselves down to a slow peaceful setting, allowing our organs to recharge and build our energy back up. This boosts the entire health of the body in every possible way.

3) Studies have shown that people who skip sleep have lower general energy and will tend to gain weight more easily. This happens for two reasons – with a lack of sleep they become tired and try to get more of their energy from food so they tend to generally over eat. And again because of this tiredness there is less energy for their digestion to properly break down the food they consume, so it leaves bigger undigested food particles behind, which eventually leads to more phlegm and fat accumulating in their bodies.

4) Sleep gives our minds a chance to calm and to quiet down. It helps them to organise and archive our thoughts and memories; and to sort out some of our hassles and problems.

It gives the mind the opportunity to be able to clear some of the clutter from our conscious minds and to reset them, preparing them to start fresh and rejuvenated again the next day.

Without enough sleep our minds can become stressed and overworked. This can lead to a lack of clarity, mistakes and bad decision making. Life can begin to seem far more complicated than it should be. Eventually without sleep, our minds can even become paranoid and delusional.

5) While most of our organs are slowing and cooling down during sleep, our hormonal ones are actually waking up and doing the opposite; they are busily producing hormones to regenerate and heal our bodies.

This happens in two phases during sleep - the first phase creates and releases growth hormones which work to replace old cells with new ones. In a healthy body any worn out old cells will be replaced during this time.

The second phase releases cortisol and other hormones to fix up and heal any damage that has been done to our cells and bodies. If we do not get adequate rest then this process is badly affected, slowing down and limiting our natural healing capabilities. With inadequate sleep we will find it much harder to recover from any physical damage or illness.

6) Our immune system runs off of our energy system. If we are tired there is less power to create white cells to defend us. Studies have shown that people who get less sleep also get more colds.

But of course our immune system does a lot more than just defend us from external bacteria and viruses. It also helps to kill and destroy anything that should not be in us. If we aren't getting enough sleep we are seriously undermining this precious system.

A lack of sleep clearly helps the mechanisms that support cancer.

Whereas all the processes that help our systems fight cancer can be boosted by good quality sleep ...

- It helps to strengthen our energy to be able to power up systems to tackle and remove phlegm and toxins from our body.
- It helps us to cool by slowing down the working engines in our bodies, letting them rest and settle down.
- It boosts the immune system, powering it up with energy to produce lots of natural killer cells to attack and remove cancerous cells.
- It helps us to quiet our minds and to lose tension and stress; thus helping to allow circulation to move more freely through the body.

If you have cancer your body will need extra rest and sleep to deal with this disease; when it slows down and becomes less active internal healing mechanisms will have a chance to come to the forefront and take charge.

So it is vital to ensure that you are getting at least eight or nine hours sleep every night. Don't attempt to skip it or to do with less. Healthy revitalising sleep is more ammunition to use to win in your battle against cancer.

Some tips for healthy sleep...

- Avoid eating stimulating heat creating foods at night time. Instead drink only water, peppermint tea, green tea and mildly bitter fruits or juices.

- Don't have your room too hot or too cold. Both of these temperatures can agitate the body and disturb restful sleep.

- Street and other sources of light are now preventing us from the natural darkness our ancestors would have had as they slept; so use blackout blinds or curtains on your window and eliminate all signs of light in the room. The darker the room is, the deeper your sleep will become.

- Develop a wind down routine for bed... Get into bed clothes and prepare yourself for sleep about half an hour before you go to bed. Do quietening and calming things. This will send signals to the brain that it is time to start shutting things down.

- If you are busy working on a creative project then sometimes thoughts will keep coming into your head keeping you awake, so put a pen and paper by your bedside and use this to put your thoughts into. As soon as this is done you will find your mind is released from the cycle and can start to switch off.

- Keep your bed for sleeping in or making love in. Avoid using it for watching television or reading and so on. When your brain associates other things with your bed you may find it harder to relax in it and then have difficulty getting to sleep.

- If you cannot get to sleep then get up and drink a glass of cool water. The cold water will deplete some of the hot energy from your stomach, heart, liver and blood. This will in turn cool the blood going to your mind, helping to turn it off and making you more tired in general.

- Try to keep the same bedtime every night, including weekends. If your mind gets use to this internal setting it will very easily and automatically know to wind things down for that time.

- Make sure you have a comfortable bed. It sounds obvious and simple, but many people sleep on the same bed year after year without checking it. And as it becomes lumpy and deteriorates, so does their sleep.

- If you feel stressed, frustrated or angry, then massage your hands and feet using downward strokes away from the head and body. Also try pinching the tips of your fingers and toes (until they sting a little). This will send hot energy and blood down away from your head, allowing it to cool down and become calm. This technique can often help you to fall asleep under those stressful conditions; however it will usually take 10 to 15 minutes to drain the hot energy from your head, so you need to be a little patient with it.

- Make sure there is good ventilation in your room by leaving your bedroom door open a little or by using a wall vent. You can also open a window if it is not too cold outside. When your room is stuffy it can cause you to overheat and can also weaken the good air and energy levels in the room and in your body. Without good energy the organs keeping you asleep won't function properly and may wake you up.

- If you can't get to sleep then don't lie there thinking over and over about not getting to sleep and the negative consequences that may cause you. This will only wind you up further, making it more difficult for you to settle down. The mind tends to create more of whatever it is thinking about, so the best thing to do is to distract it by thinking of something else. If that doesn't work then get up and do something relaxing or boring until the mind slows, calms and quietens down. Then you can try sleeping again.

- Avoid arguing, overexcitement or any other strong emotional states before going to bed. That includes reading books or watching anything on T.V. that could also create the same states. Things that distress and disturb your mind will have to be dealt with by your subconscious and conscious minds when you are asleep. These can easily lead to restless sleep, vivid dreams and nightmares.

- If you are too hot or your mind is racing or overactive then make a general increase in levels of vegetables in your diet.

The minerals and heavier particles will cool and slow down hot active energy, thus calming your heart, blood and head. Beetroot and green leafy vegetables are quite good for cooling the blood and promoting sleep.

To treat sleep problems always think of the bigger picture of your overall health in all areas - physical, mental and emotional. Concentrate on a generally healthier you and you will find that your sleep starts to improve alongside your overall well-being.

Chapter 26

The Right Type Of Exercise

Eastern traditions and medicines strongly separate from the West on their views of what are the right types and amounts of exercise we should be doing to keep ourselves in the best of health.

For the last several thousand years the Chinese have been studying the effects of exercise on the body over people's entire lifetimes. They don't just look at a short term effects like physically toned or bulging muscles, but at what happens if you continue that way of exercising over a long period of time.

The conclusions they have come to are very different to the short term Western viewpoint...

They see no difference between strenuous exercise and being overworked as a labourer on a farm, a soldier in the army, a coal miner or some other intensive form of manual work. This can often drain the life out of an individual, eventually leading to more weaknesses and illnesses, premature ageing and an early death.

They believe that doing too much exercise and doing more intense exercises like running and aerobics can be unhealthy for the body and mind. They feel too much exercise uses up and weakens resources such as energy, nutrients and hormones in the body, taking them away from the organs that need them to stay healthy and strong.

Over exercise can cause the following negative effects on the body...

1) It can deplete levels of nutrients in your blood. It can do this by using up nutrients as fuel during the exercise itself. Then afterwards it uses up blood and nutrients to repair the damage to your muscles that was caused by the strenuous activity.

As blood is directed away from the major organs and instead into recovering muscles to repair them, this has the effect of leaving those main organs in a deficient weaker state, often lacking in the resources they require to keep the mind, mood and body healthy.

Blood can become so deficient that periods in female athletes can become irregular or even stop altogether.

On the outside, the muscles are becoming bigger, more defined and toned; but internally the organs are paying the price for this.

2) When you over exercise you are basically tearing up your muscle fibres. The body releases growth and other hormones to rebuild them. This is how they are toned and strengthened up. If you continue to over exercise and to deplete your hormones it can lead to serious consequences....

Firstly just like blood and nutrients, these vital hormones are directed to muscles and away from the brain and other important organs.

And secondly, if you persist over long periods in continually demanding more and more hormones to repair and rebuild muscles, you will find that eventually the adrenal glands and other important hormone creators tire themselves out. With this exhaustion they lose their power to create the necessary hormones to run, repair and keep the rest of the body healthy.

With continuous hard exercise, physically the appearance of the body may in some ways look strong, but you will find in other ways over time the body is actually becoming weaker and weaker.

3) The mind can also be badly affected by too much exercise. When levels of energy, blood, nutrients and hormones have fallen (or have been redirected away from feeding the brain to repair muscles) the mind begins to suffer from low moods, mood swings, anxiety and other mental issues.

4) Over exercising can burn up and squander your energy. This will have a general detrimental effect everywhere in the body as organs have less power to accomplish their jobs.

But also very importantly this will leave your immune system weakened, with less ability to create killer cells to destroy external and internal bugs, and to clean up diseased and mutated cells.

Studies have shown that athletes are more likely than the general public to catch colds and even to pick up serious infections like M.R.S.A.

However in Asia they also believe that doing no exercise at all is equally as bad as doing too much. If you do nothing at all, then organs start to become lazy and the wrong things (like phlegm, fats and toxins) can start to slow down and accumulate in the system. This could help cause the body to become blocked up and stagnant on the inside, which in turn can lead to further accumulation and rotting.

So the Chinese advice is to do moderate exercise. This gives you the best of both worlds – the good benefits of exercise without any of the problems caused by under or over exercising.

Gentle movements and light exercises will help to break up stagnation and encourage circulation. They squeeze and push vessels and organs, forcing things (like blood, fluids, nutrients, phlegm, fats and toxins) that are lying in them to be moved through.

During exercise the heart pushes the blood faster, creating a forceful cleansing pressure throughout the vascular system.

On inhaling, the lungs pull purifying and strengthening oxygen into the bloodstream and cells; this empowers them and fills them full of energy. And on exhaling, the lungs push and expel fluids and waste out of the body.

The pores also open and sweat fluids and waste out through them.

All of this helps prevent phlegm and toxins gathering and adhering to cells were they can cause damage.

The right types of exercise...

If you ever visit China, you will notice that the parks are filled with people in the early hours of the morning. In them you will see the people perform many different types of activities. Above all else they love to do moderate and gentle exercises. You won't see many sweaty and strained faces or puffing and panting individuals among the crowds. The Chinese exercise more frequently with less intensity; spending thirty minutes to an hour doing more easy going, less strenuous movements.

These moderate activities do many things in the body... (**1**) They help to move the circulation ridding phlegm and toxins from it. (**2**) They tone and strengthen the muscles and make them more flexible and agile. (**3**) They help to circulate blood, oxygen and hormones up into the brain, refreshing it and giving it a boost. (**4**) They encourage the mind to focus on the movements, which can distract it, giving it a break from everyday anxieties and problems. (**5**) The movements open the lungs, allowing them to rid waste and pull more oxygen into the body. (**6**) They aid the digestion by helping to physically squeeze waste down through the intestines. (**7**) They invigorate and stimulate the adrenal glands to produce a small amount of hormones into the blood stream. And (**8**) they gently create (through the method of movement and increased oxygen intake) more energy in the body.

The key factor to understand here is that these moderate

exercises are giving you all the benefits of harder exercising without the drawbacks. They won't burn and use up all your energy, leaving you tired and worn out after them. Or leave your organs weak and unable to function properly. Or your immune system left without power to build white cells if they are needed to defend you. And they won't leave your body and muscles damaged the next day; so there is no chance of these ripped tissues stealing and draining all your blood, nutrients and hormones away from your organs, where their use is far more beneficial and productive to your overall health.

The other big benefit of this style of exercise is that because it is simply less draining than intense exercise, you are more likely to stick with it and not be put off by the pain usually associated with the harder exercises. **Moderate exercises are very easy to do and can be enjoyable and stimulating to both the mind and the body.**

The amount of exercise needed can change from one person to another. If you have an active job you need less. If however you have a sedentary job (like working behind a desk all day long) you will obviously need to do a bit more. Also if you are sick save your energy to treat the illness and don't exercise too much until you are on the road to recovery.

In general about 60 minutes a day of moderate movement is a good level to aim for. This sounds like a lot, but it can be spread throughout your entire day and can include such things as brisk walking to work or to shops and so forth.

Try to make exercise fun and do as many things that you enjoy as possible - like walking, hiking, gentle cycling and dancing.

Also try leaving the car at home for short journeys or try cycling to work. And do simple things like taking the stairs instead of the elevator; or parking the car at the furthest end of the car park away from your destination. Or getting off the bus a stop or two early and walking the rest of the way. Or if you like animals you could get a pet dog, they will get you out for lots of walks and give you good company too. Even tasks like mowing the lawn and general gardening can provide you with good exercise.

You can also simply stand up in front of the television while you are watching a program and then step up and down on the spot for about thirty minutes. If it is a good program your mind will be engaged and you will hardly notice the time fly by until your exercise has been completed. Or you could even put some lively music on and dance around your house for half an hour.

So as you can gather from reading this chapter, moderate exercise can be very helpful in both the prevention and treatment of cancer. It will push phlegm and toxins from the body and clear its internal pathways. It will flood the body with energy providing oxygen, which will help to power up cells and organs in their everyday duties. In particular it can help the immune system fight cancer by providing it with clean oxygen energy to produce more natural killer cells. It can also flood the mind with oxygen to give it a boost and to keep the mood sparked up with energy.

Chapter 27

The Weather – Our Friend And Our Foe

In the past the weather played a substantial part in impacting upon people's health. You can imagine how difficult it must have been for someone who lived 1 or 2 hundred years ago to suffer from an illness like the flu in the middle of a harsh cold winter. Living in a cold poorly heated house, it would have been very difficult to get the energy needed in the immune system to create white cells to fight off the flu or even an ordinary common cold. Or imagine how hard it would have been to get rid of a lingering chesty phlegm filled cough, living in an old damp house in the countryside during a freezing and wet winter.

Suddenly little illnesses could turn into big life threatening ones; particularly for the elderly, or for people with pre-existing conditions or weak constitutions. You can envision also working out on the land day after day in the wind or the rain; or standing on cold stone floored factories at the turn of the century, the cold could get into your system and create a chill right in to your bones.

Nowadays, we are not so vulnerably exposed to the climate. We have radiators and central heating to keep us warm in winter; and air conditioning to keep us cool in the hot summer months. Because of this, many of us have become complacent and unaware of just how damaging the weather can be. Even if we are no longer exposed to the extremes, we can still be badly affected by them.

Cold weather ...

Cold is at its most obvious in winter but it can happen at any time; the seasons of spring and autumn are often changeable and can have sudden cold spells. Returning from a trip in a hot climate to a cooler one can also compromise the body. In fact any sudden drop in temperature (from whatever circumstance) can have a strong impact on the internal workings of our systems.

Heat and cold can be seen in very simple ways... when something feels hot it is also giving out energy to its surroundings, whereas if something feels cold then it's taking energy from the environment into it.

In simplest terms - the cold weather steals energy from a hot warm body.

This is why it is paramount to protect yourself from the cold. Cold will deplete your body's power, weakening and slowing the movement and functioning of all your parts inside of you.

Most people feel weaker in the cold weather of wintertime. They often want to sleep more and do less. It is quite natural to feel like hibernating in the cold (just as we see animals do in nature). Instead the modern human being is forced to ignore these internal signals and to continue working, socialising and living as if our bodies were behaving exactly as they did in summer and there were no major weather changes occurring.

The cold will affect you in several negative ways...

(1) General tiredness – with a lack of energy all parts of the body will run less effectively on a lower power setting producing a sluggish performance.

(2) As there is less internal bodily heat to burn up and dry, and less power to push and expel, our systems will generally allow more fluids to gather and build up. If this happens excessively, then this can block internal pathways and interfere with the removal of phlegm, toxins and cancerous mutated cells from the body.

(3) As we often see towards the end of winter, people's moods can have darkened and dropped considerably. As time and the cold reigns on, minds can lose their spark and vibrancy, spiralling down into a low sullen mood. If you are battling cancer it is very important to keep your mind and willpower strong.

(4) Our immune systems run off of our energy; and as the cold robs our energy, our immune power becomes less and less, leaving us vulnerable to colds and infections.

(5) And also leaving our immune system with less ability to make killer cells to mop up and wipe out mutated cancerous cells.

So what to do...

(1) The first thing is obvious and simple... We need to wear lots of clothes, wrapping ourselves up as warmly as possible; keeping all that energy inside of us and not letting it escape out into the cold surroundings.

Forget about following fashion - your health is far more important; so wear thick hats, scarves, gloves, thermal underwear, long johns or whatever it takes to keep you warm.

(2)   If it is very cold outside then avoid making any unnecessary trips; particularly in rainy windy weather or in icy snowy conditions.

(3)   Avoid going outside or going to bed with wet hair. Cold has a tendency to lodge in dampness, making it much cooler and more damaging to the body.

(4)   Introduce more warming and heat creating foods in to your diet. Such as garlic, ginger and other mild spices; organic sugar, honey, dark teas, coffee and chocolate; and small amounts of chemical free alcohol, like an organic wine or pure vodka mixed in fruit juice. Have these stimulants with food so they have something to burn up as their fuel to create energy and heat.

They will put some warmth back into your body; but be careful - our objective is to balance the body, not to swing it from being too cold to instead being too hot. So add small extra amounts to your meals just until you feel your energy has come back and you are feeling warm and strong again.

(5)   Avoid doing too much physical, mental or any other type of draining work in cold or any other extreme type of weather.

Don't squander your energy; but instead keep the power in your organs, mind and body to keep them working efficiently and healthily.

(6)   Be careful of taking hot sun holidays in the middle of winter. Although it seems very appealing, it can throw your body out of its natural balance.

Take extra care on your return as our bodies are unable to adjust environments quickly, which can leave them caught off guard and open to catching colds, flus and other infections. So for three weeks on returning from a holiday make sure you are overprotected from any cold weather.

The wind...

The wind is a very dangerous element (nicknamed the spearhead of 100 illnesses in Chinese Medicine).

It tends to increase and drive the other types of weather deeper into us. In summer it can push the heat against our skin, drying it out more quickly. With the cold winter it can push intense cold against us constantly, pushing deep into our pores, quickly draining heat, energy and life from our bodies.

So always try to avoid drafts and exposure to the wind; if you have to go out in to it then make sure the body is well covered, wrapped up and protected from its harshness.

Heat and the sun...

The sun can be both our friend and our enemy. We will discuss the negative side first...

(1) Too much sun can burn our skin; damaging it, causing us to age quicker, and mutating cells which may lead to skin cancers.

The solution - Don't allow yourself to get sunburnt. Don't stay uncovered in the sun for any longer than that which would produce a slight change in the colour of your skin (that is if you can see it start to turn a like pink then immediately cover it up).

(2) Overexposure to the sun or heat can also dehydrate us; reducing the fluids in our bodies, damaging our blood and other vital liquids.

The solution - Make sure you drink more water, green tea and fluid filled fruit and vegetables in periods of prolonged hot weather.

(3) If the body gets overheated (with or without the sun) and if you have too many fats, phlegm and toxins within it, then these will begin to stew, cook, ferment and rot. All these putrefying fluids will congest the organs and even the mind, leading to many problems for them. Including producing an environment that would help to feed cancerous cells.

The solution - If you are overheated then (until you cool down) avoid any heat producing foods like coffee, sugar, bad fats, spices and alcohol. Instead consume plenty of green tea, white tea and bitter fruits and juices like pomegranates, plums, berries and grapes. Cooling and cleansing peppermint tea can also be helpful here too.

Now we come to the good side of the sun...

The sun can be a great friend; even if we are not directly under its shining light we can still benefit from it. It vibrates, warms and energises particles of the same air we are breathing into our bodies. This free energised air gives us more vitality and a boost to the health of our systems in summertime.

When we sit, stand and move under the suns' warm rays we also get another massive free lift to our health. Just like everything else (whether its plants in nature or man-made solar panels) the sun charges us up, filling us with life enhancing energy; giving us more power for our organs to run effectively and to clean themselves and the pathways in our bodies. And more power for our immune systems to produce natural killer cells to fight and destroy any mutating cancerous cells.

There have been hundreds of Western scientific studies showing the benefits of the sun and vitamin D. In Western terms, the suns' power is stored in us through vitamin D (a steroid like hormone). These studies have shown that with proper levels of vitamin D and sun exposure, there are decreases in many types of illnesses, decreases in premature deaths and even decreases in many types of cancers.

If you have cancer the sun will help you immensely in your fight against it, but don't let yourself get burnt or stay out uncovered in it for too long.

Western researchers say we need only expose our faces and bare arms for about 15 to 20 minutes, 4 to 5 times a week, to start to create and store plenty of vitamin D in our bodies.

You can also get vitamin D through ingesting foods such as liver, oily fish, eggs and sun-dried mushrooms; but these doses are relatively small in comparison to what the sun can provide you with - in just a short period of time.

The sun also provides energy through its infra-red rays, so even if you are covered from head to toe, these powerful rays will still penetrate into your body and provide it with free heat and energy.

So for a healthier you, make sure you spend some time outside in the sun and hot weather, and take advantage of all it has to give.

Chapter 28

How To Avoid The Common Cold

Western Medicine sees colds very differently to the way that Chinese Medicine sees them; in the West they believe that colds are solely to do with exposure to bacteria and viruses.

Whereas Chinese Medicine believes that if a bug is really virulent, then many people may succumb to it and become infected. **But in most cases for ordinary bugs that create common colds, the internal strength of the body (in particular the energy), is far more important to prevent them. If your energy is very strong you may be even able to avoid getting them altogether.**

I can personally attest to this, as a practitioner of medicine I am constantly exposed to all types of germs yet rarely get an infection. Before I studied Chinese Medicine I used to get 3 to 4 colds a year. But since I began following its techniques and practicing Qi Gong, I now hardly ever get any. And if I do it is always because I have failed to follow the theories correctly or that I was lazy and had skipped over my Qi Gong training for a period of time. So even from my own personal experience I know that **catching colds is more about the strength of the energy inside of us than exposure to germs.**

It is a fact that there are far more bugs present in our environment in summer than in winter. They breed far more easily in summer heat. They are just like flies and bigger bugs which you see swarming in hot and damp areas. And yet people generally get colds in winter, not in summer. So why does this happen? It is as the Chinese claim simply to do with the strength of your body's energy rather than the exposure to bugs.

In the cold weather your body gets drained of its energy. There is

111

not enough of it to properly power up and run your immune system. The immune system always has some white cells active in the body searching for intruders. When the white cells find some, alerts are sent back to the immune system which then goes into a massive production of more white cells. It creates an entire army full of them which are formed to hunt and kill the invaders.

So in summer, because of the heat you naturally have plenty of energy and this army is easily made. But in winter, if you have been standing out in the cold, the wind or the rain, then your energy levels have been drained. Cold will literally steal the life force from your body, and your immune system will have insufficient power to make any army to defend it. The attacking bugs will then simply walk in and set up camp inside of you.

Many of the symptoms of a cold are not actually caused by the bugs themselves who just want to feed off your body, but are created when your body tries to gather all its existing energy into your immune system, which leaves your circulation and other organs working very ineffectively.

For example, when your digestive system loses its power it will be unable to break down food properly. This leaves more waste and thicker particles behind. These get pulled through your blood, up into your lungs, where they start to congest them. Your weakened lungs don't manage to successfully breathe out these heavier particles, which causes phlegm to build up in them and their openings - the sinus cavities and the nose.

The best thing to do to avoid catching colds is daily practice of Qi Gong. It brings your energy to such higher levels that most people who practice it, will be invulnerable to colds and infections. However, if you have not the time or patience to practice Qi Gong, then these other methods to keep your energy strong and protect you are often quite successful...

(1) Firstly, stay warm... When you are warm, you will have reasonable levels of energy in the body. When you get cold they get depleted. In winter always wrap up warm. Wear extra clothes - leggings, gloves, woolly scarves and hats can all hold energy and heat in your body, vastly reducing your likelihood of colds.

(2) Avoid anything that really depletes your energy in cold weather. This includes things like over working and Western style exercise.

(3) Grief, disappointment and sadness can all have a detrimental effect on your lungs, collapsing them and drooping your shoulders. This reduces your ability to breathe and receive the energy you need from the air, leading to reduced power and ability in your immune system. Practice proper posture and the breathing techniques discussed later on in the book to alleviate this.

(4) Next up, avoid phlegm producing foods; these can block up your body and waste the precious energy it needs to run the immune system. The phlegm itself can also create great breeding and feeding grounds to harbor bacteria in.

By simply giving up dairy products you will find a reduction in the number of colds you get each year. You will also find that you will get less mucus in your nose, sinus and chest; and colds will not last as long as they would normally do.

(5) Any foods that create heat and energy are useful in preventing and dealing with colds. But don't overuse them, as this can lead to problems and illnesses from excessive internal heat. Studies on alcohol, spices like garlic and hot herbs like ginseng, have shown that the participants taking them get colds less frequently than those in the studies who did not consume them.

Actions to take if you think you are getting a cold...

If you do feel a cold coming on in winter then...

Get as much rest and sleep as possible. Avoid working and any strenuous activity which will drain away energy from the immune system.

Keep yourself warm and avoid any exposure to energy draining cold weather.

Every few hours, take <u>small amounts</u> of hot drinks like coffee and alcohol to give your energy a boost (but don't take too much or you may overheat your system).

Spicy dishes can be helpful as well. They will provide energy and also help to expectorate and push the germs out of your body.

Avoid phlegm creating fluids like dairy and hard to digest rich foods. Reduce cold and damp creating foods like water and even bland vegetables and sweet fruits until you feel well again. Any excess of fluids will have the effect of piling up in your system and creating more mucus.

However, bitter fluids like pomegranate, bitter berries, grapefruit and lemon mixed with water, can be helpful with a cold. Although these juices are cooling in nature, they are also good at purging unwelcome guests from the body. The bitterness in these juices helps to attack the bacteria, preventing it from getting a foot hold in your body and quickly forcing it out of you. During a cold, always heat the juices up or add hot water from the kettle to them (otherwise the cold juice will steal energy from you).

Follow the procedure above for a cold, but if you have a **hot fever** then it is important to use different guidelines to balance the body; so eliminate heating foods like coffee, spices and alcohol. And also increase your intake of bitter, cleansing, cooling and moistening foods like cool or room temperature lemon and water; pomegranate and any other types of fruits and juices.

Chapter 29

Chemicals And Environmental Pollution

Many claims have been made about the safety of chemicals that are being used in our environment and the increasing use of electromagnetic energy in modern technology; unfortunately these claims are often being made without the necessary scientific studies being carried out to prove they are risk free.

Everything from GM foods to signals from Wi-Fi and mobile phones to plastics covering our foods to nanoparticles and so on, these are all being labelled by their profit driven manufacturers as being perfectly safe.

In reality what is actually now happening in our world is that the human species has become part of a massive laboratory test - we are now the guinea pigs in the experiment; and if the dramatic escalation of illnesses and the deterioration of general health that we have witnessed in the last 20 years is anything to go by, then this will not end well for us.

So once again, just like I wrote about in the chapters on food, my advice is to err on the side of caution and to simply avoid as much unnatural man-made pollutants in your environment as you possibly can.

Let's now take a quick look at some of these unnatural pollutants which may be having a negative impact on your health and also may be causing damaging mutations to your DNA...

Electromagnetic fields...

In Chinese medicine Qi energy runs our bodies and minds. For thousands of years it has been seen to give the energy that creates and maintains our physical forms. But this is not just so in Chinese Medicine; quantum physics also views the world this way, suggesting that everything physical in our universe is really composed of atoms vibrating at different frequencies to cause physical forms. Even in Western Medicine, they acknowledge the electrical energy that causes our hearts to beat, the energy that runs through our nerves giving us the ability to feel and the mass of energy whizzing through our brains giving us the ability to think.

Unfortunately modern technology (be it Wi-Fi, mobile phones and their masts, power lines, TVs and other electrical gadgets) is impacting on and interfering with our bodies electrical fields. It is unclear at this time how severe this threat is; but for example the use of mobile phones in children has now been linked to increases in occurrences of brain tumours; and phone masts and towers have also been linked in multiple studies to increases in cancer for those who are living near them.

In today's age, since everyone is now online and using mobile phones, it would be very difficult to give up this technology; so instead of total abstinence, I would recommend limiting its use to essential activities.

Don't use the Internet as a pastime for just filling empty time, instead use it when you have a purpose in mind and turn it off when the job is completed.

With mobile phones, use them when you need to make a call but avoid talking about trivial matters and wasting your time on them. Rather than holding the phone at the side of your ear and brain, try to make calls using speakerphone when you can. Also avoid carrying them around in your pocket - try instead to keep them at a distance from your body, away from interfering with your body's natural electrical field.

The same also applies to any unnecessary electrical equipment in your house. If it doesn't need to be on then unplug it. In general keep electrical objects which are producing electrical currents and fields away from your personal space; for example - don't charge a mobile phone on your bedside table when you are sleeping, and keep plugged in electrical clocks away from you too.

Rather than putting a laptop on your lap - use a plugged in PC which at least gives you a little more space away from it. The same is true for TVs - sit further back from them. If you can create more space between yourself and plugged in electrical items - then do so.

Nano technology...

This involves the manipulation of molecules to make new materials and to give them new properties. Nanoparticles, created from this process are ultra tiny fragments with diameters of less than 100 nanometres. A nanometre is the equivalent of one millionth of a millimetre. They are used in many products - from silver particles placed in socks to keep your feet cool and less sweaty, to being in cosmetic creams and suntan lotion to make them less visible and easier to apply. It is estimated that as of 2010, there are somewhere between 300 to 600 products on the market place using this new technology.

The concerns that are raised here come from the fact that companies have been allowed to put these products out for our use without the necessary studies required to prove their long term safety. Currently there are no government regulations in place to protect the consumer. And alarmingly independent scientists who have started to study nanoparticles in products like sunscreen and some diesel fuels, have found serious issues which could possibly endanger our health.

They have found evidence that these ultrafine particles have moved from the skin and lungs of animals, to all the way throughout their bodies, with some particles eventually lodging in their brains. Because the particles are so small, the brain does not seem to have an efficient mechanism to remove them. There is speculation that in human beings these particles could play a role in neurodegenerative diseases such as Alzheimer's and Parkinson's.

They may also help to add to the phlegm blocking up your system and perhaps they are even damaging and polluting your cells; so it's best to err on the cautious side and avoid any products containing this new technology until it has been scientifically proven safe.

Air pollution...

We have all seen the plumes of smoke coming from giant towering chimneys in factories, or the smoky emissions spluttering from the exhaust pipes at the backs of cars and buses.

All you need to do is take a breath of this foul air to know (as you choke up) that it is very bad for your lungs and health.

Again we can't do too much about this (except maybe avoiding any unnecessary journeys into areas of high traffic).

We can however, change and control the environment in our homes and the places we work in... We can open windows to rid stale air and use air filters, ionisers and ozonators to clean the air and fill it with fresh energised particles. It's also a good idea to avoid using chemicalized perfumed air fresheners - they may smell good and hide unwanted odours, but that's no good if the bad smells are being replaced by dangerous chemical irritants. If you need your house to smell nice then you can create your own fragrances from organic essential oils and herbs or get some fresh flowers - they will release nice scents and brighten up your mood too.

Also avoid the chemical fumes released from new carpets, furniture, fresh paint and so forth; **if it smells then avoid being in the same room as it**. When you buy new things that may have been treated with chemical products then make sure you air them out - open doors and windows until the smell is gone. You can also use ozonators, which create cleansing ozone that will destroy and remove fumes and smells from the air; or even try peeled onions which astringe and pull bad odours into them.

Chemicals...

We have become surrounded by chemicals in our modern world; they are simply everywhere. It is estimated that over 75,000 new chemicals (most of which have not been tested for safety) have been introduced into our environment since the Second World War. They can be found in industrial processes, cosmetics, cleaning agents, foods, packaging, plastic, paints, furniture and other man-made products. Many of these chemicals have been linked to cancers, birth defects, neurological problems and multitudes of other illnesses. Some chemicals have been banned, but most others have not. Unfortunately, it seems only after many people have become sick (and the damage is already done) that governments start to pay attention, take the right action and finally protect the citizens who elected them.

There are far too many chemicals to list here, so below are just a few examples of suspect products containing chemicals that have been linked to causing harmful illnesses in human beings...

Plastic food and water containers - Some plastics have been highlighted to be causing serious problems in the body, particularly in the area of hormones. They can be found in water bottles, food packaging and in a coating lining the inside of tins and cans. The molecules in these plastics can literally dissolve into the food or drink that they are containing. This is exacerbated if the product is heated in the container, as molecules become much more active and disperse more easily when heated.

Pesticides and weed killers – They are commonly used to kill unwanted weeds; but guess what? Their chemicals are good at killing and poisoning other natural things (like human beings) too!

Cosmetics - These can contain a mix of hundreds of different chemicals. Perfumes, hair dyes, make up, deodorant, shampoo and everything else you put onto your skin can often leech through into blood vessels and be passed around the inside of your body.

Cleaners, laundry products and dry-cleaning – All can contain a barrage of highly potent dangerous chemicals. Many people can feel the irritant effects of these chemicals by simply walking through an aisle of these products in the supermarket - their noses and eyes can often sting from the vapours leaching from the boxes containing them.

Suntan lotions (and fake tanning products too) – Again, just like with cosmetics, the chemicals in these products can make their way through the skin and into your bloodstream where they can be passed to anywhere in the body and cause all sorts of problems.

Pharmaceutical drugs – Many of the chemicals in these do not just cause overdoses and immense harm (including death) if too much is taken, but over long periods in lower amounts can cause serious side effects and new problems for the body. Many drugs (and medical procedures – such as CT Scans) have also been linked as a cause in some types of cancers.

Teflon pans and coated cookware – Over time the coatings on these products often chip and wear away into the food they are cooking, which is then eaten, giving these chemicals a direct pathway into the body.

Insect repellents - there are many very strong unnatural chemicals used in these repellents which have been linked to causing significant problems in their wearers.

The list of chemicals and other man-made pollutants goes on and on, at this stage in the worlds development it would be impossible to avoid exposure to at least some pollutants and toxins.

But we can at least limit this exposure to the barest minimum, so …

(1) **Use electrical equipment sparingly** and when you can keep a distance away from it (such as sitting further back from your TV and so forth). Also don't chat unnecessarily on mobile phones and don't sit for hours hopping from one time consuming silly webpage to the next on the Internet.

(2) Find natural and organic replacements... These days there are plenty of companies producing chemical free natural products which can be used for household cleaning and laundry; and others for all sorts of cosmetic applications - moisturisers, make-up, suntan lotions, shampoos, perfumes, soaps and so on. You can even find companies making things like organic pesticides and weed killers for your garden.

If you can't find items in your local store then a quick search on the internet will most likely produce what you are looking for.

(3) Use green tea and bitter fruit and juice to detox and purge chemicals from your body. Just as has been explained earlier in the book, these bitter foods will help to flush away and expel toxins and unwanted chemicals.

(4) If there is a strong unnatural smell from anything new you have bought (carpets, furniture, mattresses, new or even dry cleaned clothes etc.) **then air them out thoroughly.** Open windows and doors to let fresh air circulate; and use ionisers and ozonators to clean the air too.

If you have cancer then the cleaner your body is internally the easier it will be to remove cancerous cells from your system.

Your general health and immune system will also benefit and be stronger as they do not have to deal with the burden of all these extra chemicals agitating cells in your body.

So get rid of as much man-made pollutants out of your food, your home and your life as you can.

Chapter 30

Breathing Your Way To Better Health

When we are born our very first action is to open our mouths and gasp in air. Air is the most essential thing that our bodies need, without it we would die.

The better and deeper we can breathe, the more life we can fill ourselves with. When we breathe poorly our minds and bodies suffer, we become tired and sluggish, even sleepy. Whereas when we are revitalized by air we become awake, alert and even brimming with life.

Air and its components (such as oxygen) are energetic and explosive. We only have to look in nature at the effects of air on fire to see its power. If we blow on hot embers and coals we can make them glow with energy. Or if we use a bellows, it can be used to strongly increase and fan the flames to create a raging fire.

To the Chinese the importance of air is shown in the symbol used for Qi energy; it's made up of two parts - one is food (particularly rice) and the other is air. Food and air are the essentials for human life.

In the West, for the most part we ignore and are unaware of the massive benefits we can achieve from simply making proper breathing a part of our lives. The closest we get to deep breathing is through exercise. But this (as we have seen) has its drawbacks and can also reinforce poor and unnatural breathing habits.

Because of its multiple benefits, it would be crazy not to incorporate natural deep breathing techniques into your life. It will only cost you a little of your time, effort and patience; but it will pay you back with so much good health in return.
In particular with cancer it will have a very strong impact on the disease by …

> **(1)** **Powerfully boosting your body's energy levels, and therefore your general health and your immune system.**

> **(2)** **By helping to cleanse the blood and detox the entire body, it will help to open up all the vital pathways through your system; creating an environment where cancer cells can be attacked and removed more effectively.**

> **(3)** **A lack of oxygen itself is believed to play a key role in the creation of cancer in cells...**

In healthy cells, oxygen burns up fats and sugars to produce energy and power in every single cell to carry out whatever actions it was designed to.

In cancerous cells, there is a deficiency of oxygen getting in to them, so instead of the normal energy creating process, sugars will start to ferment inside the cell to produce some energy for it to keep it alive. As the oxygen lacking cell is not getting its full requirements of power, it is believed to revert back to a simpler form which is no longer able to communicate effectively with other cells. It is believed that groups of these wild cells start to grow uncontrollably and begin to form tumours.

So by keeping cells flooded with the right levels of oxygen, new clusters of cancers may be prevented.

Before we get to the actual breathing techniques that will greatly enhance the way we breathe, let's firstly take a look at how our lungs work ...

The Lungs ...

The lungs are like an internal extension of your skin. Inside them, they create a vast network of air passageways that resemble tree branches. These become smaller and smaller until they reach tiny alveoli air sacs (about 300 million of them) which transfer oxygen and carbon dioxide (and other wastes) in and out of the lungs and blood vessels. The lungs contain a massive surface area, about 750 square foot. That's around 35 times the surface of the skin.

Our lungs perform two major vital functions in the body...

1) **Firstly they pull in air, pass it into our blood and help with the heart to pump it around the body. The air then helps to empower and create our Qi, which provides the life force energy for our systems.**

2) **Secondly they are one of the main components of the bodies waste disposal system. Every time you exhale, you**

are getting rid of significant amounts of fluids, carbon dioxide, phlegm and other toxins from the blood. (The blood has filtered absolutely everywhere through your body, gathering toxins and waste from cells, and also holding any improper or undigested particles coming from the digestive organs).

To put it as simply as possible ... when you breathe the lungs put energy giving oxygen into your blood and then help to take away the waste from it.

You can easily see the amount being removed from your lungs by breathing on a mirror; you can quickly see the moisture that is coming from your mouth condense and build up on the glass. At the same time, with this moisture, gas particles are also being emitted into the air. You take around 15 to 20 thousand breaths every day. Now if you start to multiply that by what you see on the mirror after only a few breaths, then you can see the huge amount of waste that is being cleared from your body through your lungs.

So if you are not breathing deeply then the waste is not being removed but is instead starting to build up in your blood making it and you toxic.

Now let's take a look at breathing techniques and their background...

Abdominal and Complete Breathing...

In the West people have developed very unnatural ways of breathing (**the main one is to pull in the belly as you breathe in and actually restrict the amount of air you could get into your** lungs!). This has come about from several different reasons...

1) Firstly, we have poor posture. People are now often sitting hunched at desks while working, studying or using the internet and computers.

2) The old Western habit of bottling up emotions has also led to the lungs becoming tight and stifling the energy and oxygen as it moves through them.

As young children when we had a problem we would roar crying, throwing our arms up in to the air and letting everything go. Then we quickly got over it and would become happy again. However as we aged we were criticized, ridiculed and made fun of for crying and expressing our emotions. So rather than letting them be over and done with, we instead started to hold them inside. Storing them up, where they would cause pain, obstruction and future illness.

This rigidity from incorrect upbringing stays with some people as they travel through their entire lives.

It is very easy to spot most adults in the West when they become stressed. One of the first things you will notice about them, is that they are holding themselves tensely and barely breathing. Apart from the long term damage that this is doing, in the short term, their brain won't be able to receive enough oxygen which will stop it from thinking clearly and further escalate their problems.

3) Finally, another damaging habit we have developed that is detrimental to our ability to breathe deeply, is the fashionable obsession of having a big chest and a tiny waist. This has led many men and women to pull and hold in their abdomens while puffing out their chests. This completely impedes proper breathing and is probably the biggest cause of poor breathing habits in the West.

So what way should we breathe? Well the proper way - complete breathing, is to expand outwards both the belly and the lungs as you take each breath in. Then let the lungs deflate and drop back into place; and at the same time pull the belly back in to its original starting position.

If you look at animals, children or sleeping babies, you will quite often see their abdomen naturally move up and down in a similar fashion as they are breathing.

The benefits of Complete Breathing...

1) It increases the amount of oxygen and energy being delivered to your blood. By breathing correctly you can add extra liters of air with every inhalation. This enhances and refreshes every single part of you.
Your organs, tissues and muscles will have more power and ability to do their jobs.

Your mind, which requires the most oxygen, will feel more awake, alert and calm. This allows you more control of your emotions. You can be in charge of them, rather than them leading you.

2) Your immune system will have access to a full reserve of energy; and when the body is threatened by bugs, it will be easily able to make all the white cells it requires to successfully defend you against bacteria, colds and flu. It will obviously also strengthen its ability to seek out and destroy cancerous cells.

3) Your energy levels will be increased giving you more general get up and go. As your lungs have more capacity and can breathe more easily, you will be fitter and be able to do more. Your levels of stamina will excel.

4) As you require less energy from food this will help you to manage your body weight more effectively; you will not feel the need to eat excessively to get energy in to your system and can therefore reduce intake of calories.

   The actual massaging effect involved in correct breathing also massages the abdomen, which helps to push food down through the digestive organs and also draws energy into them. This is again good for weight loss.

5) This action also massages the kidneys, and more importantly the adrenal glands. These are the most important producers of hormones in the body. This can stimulate them, clean them and help them make more hormones to heal, regenerate and power up all parts of you.

6) This type of breathing also benefits the heart. Firstly it oxygenates the heart muscle. Then it packs blood with lots of oxygen thus reducing the amount the heart needs to get to cells, so the heart doesn't have to work as hard. And

finally through this breathing, the lungs act like a bellows forcefully pushing blood through them and around the body. Again easing the workload of the heart.

7) Lastly the other big effect from complete breathing (and one that is very important in treating cancer) is the detox effect of the full exhalation. Oxygen and energy are exchanged for carbon dioxide, toxins and phlegm in the alveoli. By breathing deeply you significantly increase the size of this exchange. This will increase the amount of waste leaving your body. It will clean your blood and all parts of you, leading to a much healthier and thriving system.

How to Breathe Properly...

The first step is to breathe through your nose for everyday normal breathing. This moistens and heats the air, so it is particularly useful in winter, (however, if you find you are over-heating, it is best to temporarily breathe through your mouth to cool yourself down and regulate your temperature). The tiny hairs in the nose also help to trap and filter, dust, toxins and other airborne pollutants.

Up next is abdominal breathing... Between your lungs and the lower organs is the diaphragm. This piece of tissue can be stretched to increase the capacity and volume of air getting into your lungs. To do this you will need to **swell out your belly as you breathe in**. This sucks the diaphragm down, massaging your lower organs and allowing more air into you.

When you breathe out, pull the belly in. This will push the diaphragm back up into your lungs, helping them to squeeze out any waste and fluids.

Until you get good at this, it is sometimes useful to practice by standing with your back against a wall. Then place your hand on your abdomen and **feel it move out as you inhale and pull in tightly as you exhale.** Over time you will find it easy to extend your belly in and out, moving it over four inches and more, every time you breathe.

Finally, when you are breathing through your nose and your abdomen is moving properly as well, you can then apply the last stage, which is to **expand your chest as you breathe in and simply let it drop back into its lower position as you breathe out.**

Now in every breath you are completely maximizing oxygen and energy intake, and expelling waste as effectively as possibly from the lungs.

You will need to practice this daily for at least five minutes. It will eventually sink into your subconscious and you will find that it adopts it as your normal everyday method of breathing. In some people this will gradually happen over a month or two, in others it may take as long as a year to perfect and retain this method. But no matter how long it takes, it will eventually deliver some great benefits so do stick with it.

Chapter 31

Smoking

One of the most damaging things you can do to your lungs and to the rest of yourself is to smoke.

Smoking puts large amounts of both heat and dangerous chemicals into your lungs. Your lungs then help to distribute this into your blood where it can pollute and harm the rest of your body.

Smoking is a stimulant and therefore burns up nutrients and other sources of fuel inside of you. It will age you, damage your skin and organs, cause you anxiety and make your mind race, and most likely prematurely send you to your grave.

The biggest threat to your health brought about by smoking is cancer. Smoking is responsible for almost 90 percent of all deaths from lung cancer (the most common form of cancer in the world). More people die from it than any other type of cancer.

However, smoking doesn't just confine itself to lung cancer, it has also been linked to playing a part in the cause of many other types of cancers as well.

If you have cancer and you smoke then you need to quit them as soon as you possibly can. I know this will be very difficult but it is absolutely essential.

If you are continuing to do the very things that most likely played a big part in causing your cancer, then it is foolish and dangerous to think that any type of medicine will be powerful enough to destroy the cancer and to stop it from returning. If you want to successfully cure cancer or any other type of illness then it is a prerequisite to firstly remove the antagonists that are causing it.

There are plenty of methods to help in giving up cigarettes...

What many smokers don't realize is that part of the feel good enjoyment of having a cigarette is simply coming from the deep inhalation of air from each long drag of the cigarette. This sends oxygen flooding up to your brain, stimulating it and calming it at the same time. By frequently practicing breathing exercises, Qigong or Yoga, you can get this same (or even a better) burst of oxygen into the brain without any of the harmful toxins.

When you are giving them up, then any time you would have usually had a cigarette you should instead spend this time taking in deep breaths for two to three minutes. This will give you a surge of oxygen in your bloodstream, and replace some of the loss of energy and high you would have received from the cigarette.

Eating high energy and nourishing foods like white rice, eggs, extra virgin olive oil, nuts and seeds will also help. This will support the mind and the body, keeping them strong while you are getting away from the cigarettes.

Small amounts of coffee, chocolate, dark teas, spices and alcohol can also be used when required if the mood and will power our beginning to run on empty and need a boost to get them back up to healthy levels.

Section 6 – Your Mind Can Help You Heal

Chapter 32

The Healing Capabilities Of Our Minds...

Methods of mastering, manipulating and controlling the conscious and subconscious minds have been written into Chinese Medicine since its beginnings, thousands of years ago.

In Chinese Medicine the power of the mind is seen as an incredibly potent force. **The mind has the ability through the medium of suggestion and belief to send signals into the physical body to make it strong and healthy or to make it weak and sick.**

You can easily imagine **when your mind is in a negative or depressed state** that your shoulders, your head and your body's posture will droop and slump. And with this everything from your concentration, to your ability to breathe, to your digestion and other parts will become sluggish; your whole system will feel tired and drained, you will be running on empty. **Your body's capabilities to heal will then be impaired.** Even the reproduction of your cells will be less efficient, causing weaker cells to be created, which in turn will cause you to slump even further and lay the grounds for possible future illnesses.

We have also seen earlier in the book how stress and tension can block up internal pathways leading to heat and toxicity, which can in turn help to increase the factors which can create and feed cancerous cells.

Whereas, when we think of the reactions caused by positive

emotions on the body we see a very different picture; for example, **when you are feeling bright and joyous,** there is an extra bounce in your step, it is like you are walking on air, topped up with exuberance and extra life. Everything inside you will be buzzing and filled with more free flowing Qi energy. Now everything is working away at its highest performance, **producing thriving healthy vibrant cells.**

So one of the best ways to increase your physical and mental health is to simply train your mind into a state of positivity; with this all your internal reactions, such as the building or healing of cells will be carried out at peak levels.

To further illustrate the power within our minds we need only look at the placebo and nocebo effects...

The Placebo Effect

Placebo and Nocebo are like big pink elephants sitting in the corner of the room, creating problems for drug makers and putting a massive dent in the theories and foundations of Western Medicine; which unfortunately has denied and ignored the effects and the power of the mind throughout most of its existence.

Placebo is used in clinical drug trials; it is where a fake dummy pill is tested against a real medication to see if that drug has a genuine ability to treat an illness. If a drug outperforms a placebo then it can be marketed for sale to the public.

The big problem for Western Medicine and drug makers is that when you give sick people fake pills that do absolutely nothing in the body, it has been found to cure them of their ills in about 30 percent of cases!

To spell this out clearly, the mind having believed that it ingested

a real active medicinal cure but in reality a useless fake pill, enacted everything necessary in the body to cure it of an infliction, all by itself. The mind through the power of its own beliefs healed the body.

Every clinical trial that has been performed has noted a substantial placebo effect. It has even been shown in studies that when people are given two pills instead of one, there is a stronger effect; and when dummy pills have been printed with a well known brand name they will wondrously work even better.

To further illustrate the real physical effects that can be created by the minds beliefs let's now take a look at the Nocebo effect...

The Nocebo Effect

With this effect people taking fake dummy pills will actually often develop side effects associated with similar real pills. Symptoms such as burning sensations, sleepiness, fatigue, stomach problems, skin rashes, vomiting, weakness, dizziness, insomnia, diarrhea, swelling, tinnitus, loss of libido and upper respiratory tract infections are just some of the side effects that are reported by trial participants on these fake pills.

In simplest terms, the mind having believed that it was taking something with dangerous side effects created those same alarming side effects in the physical body; even though what it actually consumed (a simple sugar pill) was completely harmless and incapable of causing any negative effect!

Other studies depicting the power of belief have shown that patients who think they will not survive surgery are far more likely to die during it; research has also shown that women who believed they were particularly prone to heart attacks are nearly four times more likely to die from them. And **more than 50 percent of cancer patients start to experience nausea from taking chemo drugs days before the drugs could actually physically cause that effect in the body.**

Most disturbingly are cases of patients given the wrong diagnosis of terminal illnesses. One such incident of an American patient who was wrongly told he had only months to live, duly died in that allotted time frame. The autopsy showed he was misdiagnosed, was not suffering from a terminal illness and it could come to no reasonable conclusion as to why he had passed away.

The ability of the mind is truly astounding; the more it focuses on something, the more it creates of it and grows it. Think for example of a toothache or any other pain. The more you think of it the worse it seems to throb or ache. Whereas when your mind is distracted away from thinking of the pain by something you do or by someone around you, then the more the pain seems to diminish; often nearly completely fading and disappearing into the background. (This is not to say that physical pains and other problems are all in our minds and do not really exist, rather it is just to say that our mind has the power to increase or decrease them).

So we have two choices – (1) we can induce our own placebo effect, encouraging positive thoughts and beliefs to help create and increase happiness, good health and wellbeing. Or (2) we can create a nocebo effect dwelling in the negative, seeing only despair, misery and the dark side of life; which can only encourage our bodies to become weaker and sicker.

Whichever we choose will have a profound effect on our health and our ability to overcome illness.

In the next chapters we will see how we can utilize key theories and elements of Chinese Medicine to practice and master positivity to strengthen and enhance both our mental wellbeing and our physical health too.

Chapter 33

How Our Minds Work

The mind can be split into two basic areas that produce thoughts; they are **the conscious and the subconscious minds.**

The conscious mind is the part of you that is reading and processing this sentence right now. **It thinks, computes, processes, and makes judgements and decisions. It is active when we are awake and it tries to make sense of our interactions in this world we live in.** It is fed information externally from society and its surroundings and internally from your subconscious mind and your soul.

In terms of health and wellbeing the conscious mind has incredible power through concentration, focus and repetition to establish positive programs to run in your subconscious.

Whereas the conscious mind is more like the central processing unit of a computer, the subconscious is more like the background programs that run on the computer and the data and information contained in its memory banks.

The subconscious contains all the patterns, habits and routines originally formed at birth to run your body; and formed thereafter through your life experiences and the programming

you receive from society (that is – all the brainwashing you get pushed into your mind from school, parents, religions, governments, authorities, TV, movies, fashion and so on).

These programs in your subconscious run your body and your life on auto pilot, so your conscious mind is freed up to interact with new developments.

This is just like learning to drive a car; when you start to learn how to drive your conscious mind is very aware and notices every little action. However after a while, your subconscious having created patterns from repeated actions, takes over and you seem to be able to drive with ease. Your conscious mind is then freed up and you can easily hold a conversation, listen to the radio, think of what you have to do later and of course still drive safely all at the same time.

Most of our reactions to life come from our subconscious. Even when we meet new people or do new things, references from past experiences come constantly from the subconscious into the conscious mind, prompting us to behave in certain ways in these new situations.

The problem is a lot of these prompts may not be beneficial or desirable. We may have lots of unwelcome habits now hardwired into our subconscious from negative past experiences that we have endured. These may now continually prompt us to behave in sad, angry, shy, anxious, critical, fearful, argumentative, deceitful and other unhealthy ways. We may even make judgements about people and situations not on the real current events and facts we are presented with, but on pre-judgements formed by past memories in our subconscious. This is obviously not sensible or productive in leading us towards healthy and happy lives. It often instead traps us into behavior which prolongs misery, ill health and suffering.

In terms of illness, if our subconscious expects us to be weak and sickly or if it is in a negative emotional state, then it seems to send inferior orders around our bodies and internal processes are performed poorly; this affects both our bodies ability to stay healthy and also its ability to recover from and defeat any illness.

Another common action the subconscious takes is to feed the conscious mind with whatever predominant emotions it has learnt to have most of. This means that if it has mainly been fed sadness and negativity, then even when it experiences something joyous, it quite often and quickly returns to what it knows most of, in this case negativity.

The good news is if we consistently practice optimism, positivity and healthy mental outlooks, then that is what our subconscious will eventually push forth.

When it reaches this state then even if we are currently going through a bad experience, if our subconscious has been flooded with positive thoughts it will keep pushing that into our minds instead, buoying and strengthening them up and helping us to calmly and more easily think and live our way through whatever difficult dilemma it is that we are facing.

In terms of cancer, when the subconscious is strengthened it will send superior signals and messages around the body influencing it to work at the highest levels to use all available resources to destroy and remove the cancer and prevent it from coming back.

Don't get me wrong here, when I talk about the power of the mind it may not be strong enough by itself to kill the cancer, but it is another great asset to add to our growing arsenal of weapons which will help to eradicate it.

We will talk more about the many positive things we can do to influence and retrain our subconscious minds shortly.

But to accomplish this it must be stressed that new programs and health producing habits must be reiterated over and over again into the subconscious, until they rewrite negative patterns that are stored there. After that to keep the subconscious in a healthy and productive state, it should be constantly topped up through methods such as meditation, positive affirmations and right thinking.

Chapter 34

Three Paths To A Healthier Mind...

Before we start, I would like to say that I know if you have cancer you are going through a very difficult and traumatic time, there is absolutely no question of that. Initially your mind will be very shocked and disturbed by the news of the diagnosis; in this state you will be unlikely to be in a receptive mood to want to hear how to be positive or happy. But if you can find ways to accept and to start to follow some of the processes below then this will give you a much stronger chance of defeating the cancer. It will also lessen the burden on your system, improve your general quality of life and help you recover more quickly from intense Western medical treatments like chemotherapy.

There is no question that what has happened to you is very sad and tragic, but please do not wallow in despair and hopelessness. If you do you will only weaken your body further and allow the cancer to become stronger; instead please find the strength from somewhere deep within you and turn your mind to a positive empowering attitude which will best enhance your body's ability to both survive and to thrive.

So now let's take a look at some methods that can improve the way our minds work ...

(1) Observe Your Mind and Question Your Thoughts ...

With the mind you must become its observer. You must watch and take note of thoughts and emotions as they come into your brain.

Objectively start to judge them and the responses they create throughout you and your entire body. For example, are they making you feel physically tense, shaky, tired or weak?

Are these thoughts even genuine and appropriate reactions for the situation you are in? Or are they just automatic repetitive responses coming from what your subconscious has been conditioned to believe (from past experiences or from the influences of other people and society).

Examine all the emotions as they appear in your mind; think about them logically and rationally, and question them to see if they are really in your best interests. Then after reflecting on them, decide if these thoughts are more useful or more harmful to you. **If they are not good for you then start to practice the ways described in this and other chapters to drop these harmful thoughts from your mind.**

There are two steps needed to start to remove negative thoughts from the mind – one is awareness and the other is practice.

The first step - awareness, allows us to wake up; to stop living our lives on auto pilot. It helps us to really question our thoughts, emotions and behaviors; to question what they are and where they are coming from, then to deeply understand whether they are good for us and for other people around us, or are they instead just damaging our health, our happiness and our lives.

For example, if we truly think about anger and its consequences, we need to ask ourselves do we really want to be controlled by this emotion or to have to deal with the pain that it often brings.

There is a famous saying by Buddha that holding onto anger is like holding a hot coal in the palm of your hand with the intention of throwing it at the person who is annoying you – you may hurt them but in the process you will hurt yourself too.

In nearly all cases anger won't lead to the best outcome in an argument, instead it quite often leads you to say and do things you would not if you had stayed cool and clearheaded. Later you will most likely start to regret your reckless actions, wishing you could take back what you had said.

Or how about angers effect on the other person, they often feed off the strong emotions coming from you and it gets them all riled up and aggressive as well. Now two minds are acting irrationally and all common sense and reasoning disappears.

But instead if you can control your emotions (prevent anger) and stay calm and focused you will find your mind can logical think its way out of a problem and come up with the best solutions for all involved.

However, anger is not alone, most emotions be they sadness, guilt, fear, jealousy, bitterness, disappointment or the like, only produce negative consequences and detrimental effects for both you and those who are around you. Examine them all, and with awareness, then one by one let all those negative emotions go from your mind and from your life; leaving you to embrace only the ones that actually help your body in a positive way, that is the emotions of happiness and love, they are the only ones you truly want or need.

When we drop negative emotions from our present it can also have a big impact on our past too. Our memories quite often have many emotions attached to them. For example you will have lots of past memories lodged in your brain that make you angry when you think about them. You could pay a psychiatrist a fortune to sit with you and talk you through resolving each one of them; this would also be a very painful and disturbing experience as each old memory is rehashed and felt again fresh in your mind.

But instead if you can change the big picture, the way you see and understand emotions, then your mind will begin to work in a different better way. In this case if you can resolve and change your beliefs regarding the validity of anger and how it actually harms you rather than helps you, then you will find (as you drop anger) that all past memories you are holding in your subconscious which are tainted by anger will begin to diminish; leaving only the lesson to be learned and the wisdom that was garnished from those negative experiences left behind.

(2) Be Careful What You Feed Your Mind...

When you sit down to watch television or start to read a novel, be very careful what you have chosen to take into your mind. We do not invite dangerous criminals into our homes nor do we pile junk foods into our bodies, yet **we regularly leave the doors to our minds wide open for any destructive element to infiltrate and disturb them**.

Our modern society now constantly pushes and glamourizes drama, sensationalism, conflict and perversity towards us. There are very few family orientated, heart-warming and positive TV programs or uplifting books being created anymore. Instead we have ones filled with violence, horror, degradation, sadness, immorality, cheapened and exploitive sex, wealth and greed, corruption, gossip, betrayal and many other negative aspects and emotions.

Unfortunately when we are watching these, particularly if we start to get emotionally involved, our subconscious (and imaginations) starts to absorb this presentation as if we were really a part of it.

The subconscious acts like a sponge soaking up all this negativity. If we constantly watch or read about sadness our minds will become more depressed, if we watch violence we will feel more violent, if we watch programs about gossip we will be encouraged to talk crudely about others, and so forth. Unless we observe and question our thoughts, what our minds have been fed will unconsciously seep back out of them causing harm and destruction to our health, relationships and lives.

How often have you seen a disturbing image or even heard a crummy annoying song on the radio only to have it repeat again and again in your conscious mind. Once it goes in, (unless you have a very strong mind) it is hard to get it back out; so the best solution is not to put these troublesome thoughts into the mind in the first place.

So when you are watching TV, reading or even when you are hanging out with friends, be careful what is being fed into your mind as this is what will be repeated by your subconscious and projected into your life. Just as you watch your diet and avoid eating junk food, be just as careful in preventing junk from being fed into your mind and soul. Instead choose more uplifting and positive TV and books to read.

If you are around negative people, the greedy manipulative competitive types who gossip and bitch about others, then push the conversation to more positive topics or find a better quality of people to hang out with. Otherwise those people will be planting destructive seeds of negativity into your mind which will have a detrimental impact on the relationships in your life and on the health of your body.

(3)   Dealing With Negativity And Painful Past Experiences...

Unfortunately life often seems to lack a sense of justice; bad things can seem to equally happen to both good and bad people. Those who do wrong and create pain for others have no one to blame but themselves when inevitably the consequences of their own actions come back to their doorsteps. But for those who generally live in a good way and avoid doing harm to others, life can sometimes seem very unjust and unfair. We can regularly meet selfish, inconsiderate, thoughtless and corrupt people. They can be in our families, in relationships, as co-workers in our workplaces or strangers we meet on the street; or even sometimes they can be friends who abuse our trust, let us down and turn out to be anything but friendly.

When something bad happens to us (especially in childhood when our minds have less wisdom and experience in knowing how to defend themselves from other peoples maliciousness), our subconscious will often react to pain and cruelty by trying to build a wall around our emotional hearts and souls to protect them. We end up pushing this part of us deeper and deeper inside to try to disconnect it from the cruel behaviors of other humans. The problem is, **when we close our souls off we are also closing off the ability to feel and surround ourselves in the only real and meaningful love and happiness that there is to be found in our lives.** If we have not access to our souls then we can never truly feel or know what real love, peace and joy is. Instead all we are left with is meaningless empty pleasure (such as is felt by sociopaths).

The outside world is quite good at feeding us with pleasure. However these temporary superficial highs and fixes only numb our pain and distract our minds from our real issues. Often leaving us back in the same spot (feeling empty and dead on the inside) and facing the same problems we originally had when the pleasure has passed.

On the other hand if we can manage to take down the walls around our hearts and our souls, and feed them with positivity and real wisdom then they will grow; and we will find that a genuine love springs forth from them which keeps us wrapped in a strong continuous healthy high and allows us to live our lives in a rewarding meaningful way.

The love that comes from the soul is a true and genuine sense of happiness and belonging. It is more of a feeling than a thought. It is warm, comforting, secure, peaceful and yet at the same time alive and invigorating. It is very unlike pleasure, which is a purely mental experience, giving you a boost and then dropping you, often leaving you disappointed and in a state of craving for a new experience to replace it. That is not real happiness, not even close.

The love emitted from the soul is entirely independent of all external forces outside the human-being; it does not require wealth, power, vanity or any of the other trappings of the ego to produce it. This type of love is the exact thing that all human beings need to complete and fulfil their existence. Unfortunately, most people who get caught up in the consumerism and competition of our modern capitalistic world are searching for this happiness but are looking entirely in the wrong places where it cannot be found. Instead of outside, we need to turn our focus back inside and release our souls.

This love inside is free and abundant. It takes nothing from you to create it but in turn relaxes and empowers you. Your physical health and mental well-being will thrive on it. It makes you smile, gives you bliss, makes you feel great, with it you will often find you are happy for no reason at all; it has no limits. The closer you get to real love in the soul, the closer you get to long fulfilling happiness, to creating your own personal heaven on earth.

But to do this it takes you to **free your soul**, to allow it to come back out into this often harsh world. This time however, to protect your sensitive soul (unlike when you were a child and everything you experienced got dumped into your subconscious), this time **using proper mental techniques and awareness, you will be in control and choose not only what is now allowed into your mind, but you will also reprogram what is already there; clearing away any negative emotions and past traumatic experiences which are still repeating on your conscious mind and interfering with your present day happiness and health.**

To remove the power attached to these past negative memories we must diminish any emotion attached to them. By altering our beliefs and views regarding emotions (such as anger, bitterness, disappointment, sadness and so on), this will automatically start to reduce undesirable emotions from our memories.

But in this process, we should definitely <u>garnish any wisdom or lesson to be learnt from a past experience</u>, as this will help us to make better choices in our present. From bad events we should learn and become wise, otherwise we are bound to make similar mistakes again and trap ourselves in a cycle of suffering.

We also need to forgive others in order to release ourselves from the past. This does not mean that we excuse their bad behavior, it just means we lose the hate and the anger we have for them. **For those emotions are imprisoning us and preventing us from moving on.**

If you are someone who has harmed others in the past and you are filled with guilt and shame, then you too need to let these go, they are a major burden on your mind and soul; and they our helping to prevent you from attaining real happiness and peace.

There are two steps to doing this. Firstly, you need to do all that is possible to undo the damage that you did to someone else. They may still be feeling hurt by what you did and if you can, you need to fix this.

Secondly, the fact that you have thought about what you have done, and that you feel bad about it is actually a good thing. It shows that you are genuinely sorry and that you have begun to take responsibility for your actions. So once you have learnt and grown from any past mistake, once you are now committed to positive change and will do your best to avoid repeating any problems you may have caused, then you have now evolved and become a different person, a new you. **Your mind and soul are no longer forming the same person who harmed others**. Your soul has matured and developed. So it is time to forgive yourself, move on and create a wiser happier future for yourself and all others who become a part of it.

Chapter 35

Other Positive Steps You Can Take For A Healthier Mind ...

We will start with a very simple one ...

<u>Smile</u> - Smile meaningfully as much as possible; and even when you don't want to smile, smile anyway. **A smile ignites electrical pathways in the brain which cause a calming and uplifting effect throughout the entire body.** Every time you smile you are benefiting your physical body and health.

In the same way, hold your posture upright and open; this too sends signals to the subconscious that all is well and good. In this state of mind the subconscious will carry out tasks around the body in peak performance, rather than being sluggish and disruptive.

Breathe - By having an open posture it will also enable you to breathe properly. Remember to breathe slowly and deeply, this will energize both body and mind, powering up your spirit and strengthening your positive emotions. With shallow breathing oxygen in the brain is reduced and your mind will most likely falter and panic, increasing your worries and problems.

One of the first things to be affected when you get stressed is your breathing, as your body tenses the muscles around your ribcage will seize and prevent you from inhaling properly. So consciously be aware of this and practice daily breathing techniques to re-enforce good breathing behavior. This is important for everyone to do, but is especially important for anyone who works behind a desk or at a computer.

Write It Down – One way of getting rid of garbage out of your subconscious is to simply write it down, when you do this it seems to release the damaging thoughts from your brain.

When our subconscious has an unlikeable thought that it doesn't seem to know what to do with, it has a tendency to repeat and repeat this problem. When we write it down the subconscious recognizes that we now have a written record of the issue so it simply no longer has to carry it, it then drops it from the mind.

Give this one a go, it is an easy method that will work for and relieve you of some (but not all) of your problems.

Negative Chat - Cut out the pessimism, gossip and defeatist self-talk; all these are sending very negative messages to your subconscious and will corrupt it, causing it to create poor health and even more problems in your life. Statements like, "I can't" and "it's too difficult" re-enforce weak patterns of thinking in your subconscious mind and will lead you away from your goals.

Always practice optimism and keep your mind positive. Look on the bright side of life as much as you can; look for the opportunities, not for the problems. This will help to keep you strong enough to continue on when times are difficult. If you give in to the gloom you will find it will quickly drag you and your health into the gutter.

Your subconscious mind simply grows and creates more of anything it dwells on. It does not make logical decisions but merely follows suggestions from your conscious mind. If you say to yourself "think of a red balloon", you will see an image of a red balloon pulled from your subconscious memory banks into your mind. However if you say the opposite, "don't think of a red balloon", you will still get the same result. So always concentrate on what you do want rather than on what you want to avoid or else the subconscious will just start to produce the very things you are trying to escape from.

If you consciously dwell on negativity, your subconscious will look for events within and outside of you to create more of the same. So always look for, embrace and re-enforce positivity; in your words, in your thoughts and in your actions. Otherwise your negativity will just create a self-fulfilling prophecy and bring you more of its kind.

This is one of the reasons why everyone should practice being good, because when you are concentrating on being mean or bad, in actuality you are focusing that state into your subconscious mind and it will inevitably do its best to create the same state for you that you have been creating for others. Only good sincere thoughts can manifest and bring to you the real happiness you truly long for.

By practicing and being loving, peaceful and positive this will

eventually become the natural state inside your mind. However, be positive but be wise; do not tolerate bad situations or bad people. Don't get dramatic or angry, just smarten up and move on. Take your business and kindness elsewhere, where it and you can be respected and appreciated.

Visualize Happiness - Don't just look for the positive side to an event but actively create and imagine a joyous outcome in your mind. This will get your subconscious to work in the background to find ways to accomplish this goal. It may subtlety make you behave in a different manner or push you to make a different intuitive choice to accomplish this outcome. It is much more logical to have it visualizing happiness and creativity, and working with your consciousness, rather than having it caught up in some form of negative learned past behavior which could only lead to problems for you.

This is the same for anyone who is dealing with cancer; every time you drink your green tea and eat your healthy food, every time you exercise and take deep calming cleansing breaths (and so on), you must visualize yourself getting healthier and stronger. The more you re-inforce these thoughts and empower yourself the more able your body will be to wipeout and destroy that cancer.

Lose the Fight, the Resistance, the Anger – In this world there will always be some rotten degenerate who wants to in some way steal from others; or who wants to belittle and attack them just because they are jealous of them; or simply their ugly big egos just want to show off; unfortunately it is getting more and more difficult to escape these parasitic people.

But if we get angry at them, without them even having laid a hand on us, we will have actually helped them to hurt our minds and our physical health too – when you think about that it doesn't seem to be a very clever thing for us to do. Now I am not telling you to let these people get away with these things, I am just saying to deal with them in a more intelligent way, that defeats them but that doesn't mess with your head or tie your body up in knots with damaging stress.

In a fight or argument it is always better to keep tranquil, which will allow your mind to act in the clearest and most logical manner, in order to attain the outcome you want.

It is also a good idea to try to stop fighting every little thing in your life that does not go your way. Be sure to stay true to your inner self and keep your goals and beliefs, but do change paths and move around the obstacles that life throws in front of you, rather than trying to fight them all head on. You will accomplish much more in the long run, save yourself lots of energy and avoid much frustration and heartache by following this approach.

The Past Cannot be Changed - If bad things happened to you in your past then there is no point in dissecting them over and over again, you will greatly disturb your mind and steal any peace from it by repeatedly rehashing past wrongs.

Quite often there is no valid explanation, no logic, no reasoning as to why people do bad things to us. And no matter how hard we look for justification as to why people wronged us we will never find any answers.

The simple truth is that people wrong other people because they are greedy and selfish, they simply want their own way and more for themselves no matter what the cost is to anyone around them; there is no excuse for their behavior.

So if you have been wronged then learn the lesson from the experience (which may simply be to learn how to avoid it happening again) and then drop it. Let it go, so you can move on with your life.

Live in the Present - Forget about future outcomes and past problems, instead try to create happiness and love in each moment as you are living it.

When you do things for others, forget thoughts of any future reward or compensation for what you are giving them. Lose the expectations and instead live in the love and happiness you are generating right now. That is your reward, you are already there experiencing the joyous moment, your happiness is already complete; so just slow down, enjoy it, bask in it and take it all in.

Free Yourself and Embrace Happiness in Any Form - Stop conforming to what society is telling you is hip, trendy and cool. **Make your own mind up as to what you like and stop listening to others.**

The object of life is to become happy, not to listen to the mindless who are just following the crowd. Clearly as rates of anxiety and depression are dramatically increasing it is very unwise to simply follow the crowd anymore, unless you too want to end up becoming sick and unhappy.

I wasted considerable amounts of my younger life trying to live up to the expectations of others and there often ill-informed and poorly thought out ideologies. So **break free, start enjoying what you want, not what is merely fashionable and correct in society.** The next time you buy something buy it because you like it; because its color, its texture, its shape makes you interested in it and makes you smile, not because someone has told you this will keep your standing in society as one of the so-called trendy people.

And the next time you make friends with someone, do it because you like them; not because they are the coolest people to hang out with and will make you look good in front of your peers. Be friends with them because they are nice, they are good people and forget what ranking society has given them. So many good relationships and opportunities for happiness have been destroyed because one person thought it would be seen as uncool to hang around with another. As young kids we didn't care what our friends looked like or the way they acted. We only cared about having fun with them. It was only after being bullied by society that we changed our minds. So break free and get that genuineness back into your relationships; and you will find plenty of real love and happiness comes along with it too.

Remember, health and happiness are your real goals. It is not necessary to become wealthy and successful, but only to become healthy and happy. It is not necessary to become famous and popular, but only to become healthy and happy. Always keep this thought active and conscious in your mind, follow it and you will be truly rewarded.

Do the Groundwork - You Get Back What You Give - So if you want real, honest, good rewarding relationships, then expect to put in some real effort to build up trust and strong foundations in them. If you do encourage and create genuine friendships and relationships, you will be rewarded with so much more than money can buy you.

Spend less of your time watching TV and being on the internet and more of your time building honest, good, loving, real relationships with good people; that will keep you with a smile on your face and warming love in your heart.

Do Good, Spread Love - By practicing good and promoting love, peace, happiness, honesty, wisdom, meaning and joy, we start a chain reaction of positive actions around us that will feed into society. The more we promote this, the more good will return to us and enhance our own lives. But if we promote criticism, gossip, judgement, bitterness, sourness and selfishness, then the odds are that is what will be returned to us.

You cannot go wrong by dwelling on love, peace and happiness; focus on them to bring more of the same into your life.

"Thousands of candles can be lit from a single candle, and the life of the candle will not be shortened, happiness never diminishes by being shared" - Buddha.

Chapter 36

Meditation – The Art Of Mastering The Mind ...

Meditation is a method which is used to gain control of and then to master the subconscious mind.

Most of your daily experiences are not performed by your conscious (aware, questioning, reasoning and thinking) mind but are run by your subconscious, leaving you mostly in a state of running on auto pilot.

The subconscious is responsible for controlling the physical like your breathing or your heartbeat; to automatic emotional responses pulled from past learned behavior, to facial expressions and other habits and characteristics you have formed, to speaking in a foreign language or performing any other skill you have learnt. It is basically responsible for everything your conscious mind isn't directly participating in.

The subconscious can cause problems for us in many ways …

1) If our subconscious is in a negative state and running in a poor or dismal way, it sends out orders that will produce lower quality functioning, healing and regeneration in the physical body.

   If it is filled with bad experiences and stress, then as it becomes more paralyzed by these detrimental emotions it will also tighten and seize up movement and activity in the body causing the emergence of further physical ills.

2) Another set of problems can commonly occur if it becomes overwhelmed by thoughts.

   The Chinese often then refer to the subconscious disrespectfully by calling it "the chattering monkey". It has become filled with too many worries, cares, emotions and problems.

   It will now simply become less productive and will instead start to flush gibberish and an abundance of thoughts into our consciousness, disturbing and confusing it; and preventing it from finding the peace and clarity it needs to make right decisions and steer its way out of life's problems. This can obviously lead to many problems in relationships, work and all other aspects of life.

When the mind becomes this screwed up it will undoubtedly also lead to poorer or incorrect commands being sent to the physical body leading to a down turn in its health.

3) **The subconscious is the creator, feeder and home of our ego.** The ego is a false projection of our own self-importance. It is in many ways like our own internal sociopath, but in this case **it selfishly feeds itself at both the expense of those around it and its own owner.**

The ego is always hungry and its desires can never be quenched, if one is fulfilled it is simply replaced by another, it always demands more and more, and to be better than others.

It has no soul, morals or values; it is artificial and purely influenced by external events in society. It is not useful to its owner, who it often leads in the wrong direction, dragging them into negativity, and stealing attention away from the real objectives in life. It can only create pleasure but not happiness.

It detracts power and limelight away from the person's inner real self, their soul.

Nor is it of any use to the outside world. The ego spreads criticism, greed, gluttony, competition and other negative qualities. It favors no-one but itself. When it is winning the battle against the soul, the person will not have the opportunity to experience real happiness and love. But will instead be left on a meaningless pleasure seeking rollercoaster of emotional ups and downs.

As time goes by and the enemies of the ego (such as old age, sickness and loss of power) start to win, there inevitably comes the time when the downs greatly start to smother the ups, leading its' owner into a soulless life of emptiness, lovelessness, bitterness regret and misery.

If you are to ever truly find happiness and the superior health and well-being that thrives in that state, then at some stage you must deal with the ego in your subconscious, and quite simply diminish its power and destroy it.

Meditation when practiced correctly can be a very successful method to master and control the subconscious mind and to quell the ego within it.

The objectives of meditation...

1) To bring peace and tranquility to the conscious mind so it can live in a state of calmness and relaxation.

2) To bring clarity and power to the conscious mind so it can think lucidly and achieve the best outcome in any interactions with other people or anything else in this world.

3) To quiet down the subconscious so it has less interference (from the chattering monkey!) as it does its real work of

running background tasks to keep the body working productively and in the peak of health.

4) To use the conscious mind to effectively reprogram the subconscious into working in a more effective state.

Whilst you are in a meditative trance the subconscious will be at its most quiet; this is the most opportune time to plant suggestions into the subconscious that will take firm root and start to create that effect in the body and personality.

In deep meditation you can easily program yourself in to being happier, healthier, more positive and into so many other good states.

5) To overpower the subconscious to stop it from repeating painful past memories. To instead learn the lesson from these harmful experiences and to then finally drop any painful emotions attached to them from the mind.

6) When you silence the ego, the empty space that is created is filled by your real self – your soul. The more this happens the more you will find out and understand who you really are; and what is really valuable and meaningful in this life. This is one of the reasons why meditation in the East is so linked to enlightenment.

Different types of meditation...

There are many methods and styles of meditation; when you study them you begin to see clear patterns of their common threads and of how these will cause effects in the mind.

If you want you can simply sit cross legged in the Lotus position, or you could adopt a pose from Yoga. Yoga is not just a set of stretching exercises as believed to be by many in the West, but is actually a spiritual practice. Yoga means union, and in this case to unify with God and the Universe.

My personal favorite form of meditation is through Qi Gong exercises. But if you are versed in Yoga or some other method then you can try incorporating some of the techniques shortly described (in the next chapter) into your own style of meditation.

If you are a strong follower of a particular religious faith then do not think that by practicing meditation you have aligned yourself in any way with any other type of religion.

Historically in the Christian and other Western religions, meditation has always had a strong place. Nuns and monks have always followed a similar practice through everything from vows of silence and isolation, to prayers and direct meditation. They do this to find quiet and peace in their minds, to allow deeper clarity and connection with their souls and with God. In the East nearly every religion, be they Buddhist, Taoist, Hindu or so forth, uses meditation also for this exact same purpose. So do not have any fear that you are betraying your religion by following any of the meditative techniques in this book.

They are just simply good techniques to allow you to have more control of your own mind. From this book you can take whatever techniques you find beneficial and apply them to your own religious beliefs.

If you are an atheist or have some other form of belief then meditation will also only benefit you; by increasing the energy and power in your brain allowing it to function more calmly and clearly, therefore helping you to make better and more productive decisions in your life, and thus allowing it to be more successful and fulfilling.

Chapter 37

Reprogramming The Subconscious Mind ...

In this chapter we will discuss implanting suggestions into the subconscious mind and leading it to a better state of health.

To alter programs, behavior and memories in our subconscious, we firstly need to quieten and subdue it. **The more we can turn it off, the more we can get it to listen to our suggestion.** So just like in a hypnotic trance, try to go into a deep state of quiet and calmness (and turn off that chattering monkey). You will find that your conscious mind has a much stronger and more successful ability to implant suggestions into your subconscious in this state.

Through focusing we also strengthen our conscious mind, we empower it and give it control; again this enables it to be better able to rewrite the subconscious mind. Anytime we focus on just one thing, such as breathing, a candle or a spot on the wall then we are pushing energy into our conscious mind and making it more powerful.

Next up we can use imagery, visualizations and word associations.

As we are living our lives our subconscious is recording and interpreting everything in the fore and backgrounds. It starts to associate positivity with light, warmth, white, gold, sunshine, angels, heroes, success, vibrancy, happiness and so on; it also associates negativity with darkness, cold, boredom, pain, sadness, suffering, demons and villains etc.

So in our subconscious minds we have developed a history of good life affirming words and images; things that will light up the subconscious, making it run well, producing health and joy in the body. And also negative soul destroying words and images, causing the subconscious to slow, falter and produce ill health.

When we are meditating, practicing Qi Gong or Yoga, we should only utilize these positive images and word associations to emphasize our desired results to the subconscious.

Quite often a striking visual image of health and power can have a greater more pronounced effect on the subconscious than just telling it to get healthy, (so creating positive healthy images in your mind's eye can help you succeed in your goals).

When you are meditating on words and images, make sure you attach positive happy emotions and feelings to them. If you were to send a message like, "I will have a successful interview tomorrow", while you are feeling nervous and fearful, then the subconscious will get confused signals and will be unable to generate success and stability in that interview. Likewise if you instruct your body to be healthy while you're feeling angry or sad, you are most likely to throw a spanner in the works and produce a poor or low quality outcome.

If you find it difficult at the beginning stages, to summon up any real happiness when you are pushing a positive affirmation into your subconscious; then just smile as you say the affirmations to yourself.

So while meditating use lots of positive visualizations, bright life affirming and spiritual images, and mood enhancing words. You can take a word like happy and while repeating it in your mind, think of the feelings you get when you are happy. You will find by repeating this word you will induce this state in yourself. The next time you are in a negative situation you can say this word in your mind, and the association in your subconscious if it has been implanted repeatedly will immediately start to cause changes in the body to recreate these feelings and then change your mood.

You can apply different words in your meditations to induce different states of mind. Such as happy, relax, release, health, strength, power, peace and love etc. Just repeat these positive images and feelings into your subconscious and you will eventually find that you are creating a permanent state of positive well-being and health in your mind; the subconscious will then start to recreate the same in your body.

Outside of your meditations you can also create positive affirmations for your mind by surrounding it with symbolism that promotes love, happiness, and tranquility; everything from positive religious statues, to soothing colors, to lucky charms and talisman. All of them will have a subtle and influential impact on the health of your mind and body. If you imagine that you are in a room with a smiling Buddha statue, you are obviously less likely to feel angry and so forth; **so ensure for your good health to surround yourself with positive imagery.**

You can even write positive messages on sticky pads in key areas around your home, car or work place. When seeing these affirmations they will refocus and inspire your mind towards its goals.

Be aware, that if you do the opposite and surround yourself with dark, violent, sad or oppressive imagery or music, then that is what your subconscious will focus on and try to generate in your actual life. This will not bring you the happiness you desire, but will instead ultimately lead you towards more suffering and pain. So be cautious in the choices of what you are allowing around you and

165

encouraging into your mind.

This also includes many of the chat shows, soap operas and programs that we now watch on the TV, or in films we view in the cinema. These are being viewed by two minds in you, the conscious which is seeing them just as entertainment and the subconscious which sees them more so as instructive. When they are portraying negativity, such as gossiping, arguing, betrayal, despair, hatred and so forth, then all of that is being absorbed (but not logically filtered) by the subconscious, which will in turn try to recreate events in your life to bring them or similar experiences to you. Just like the way the subconscious will bring you the red balloon even if you don't want it, as we discussed earlier in the book. **So be very careful what you watch and invite into your mind.**

Section 7 – Qi Gong

Chapter 38

Qi Gong – The Art Of Superior Health…

What is Qi Gong ?

Qi Gong is the art of cultivating energy. It is usually performed as a set of moving and standing exercises which also incorporate breathing techniques and meditation. **Its aim is to increase the amount of energy in the body, mind and spirit.** Obviously with more energy, all internal systems to keep the human being in peak health and strength will be empowered up to work at superior levels.

Qi Gong is thousands of years old and forms part of the roots and foundations of Chinese Medicine. Historically it has been used in three main areas; they are healing, martial arts and spiritual progression.
In medicine it is used to build, heal and manipulate energies which control the physical body and mental and emotional welfare. It is commonly used in Chinese hospitals in the treatment of cancer and many other conditions. In martial arts it is used to create power, speed, skill, agility, alertness and strength for combat. It also provides lots of power for improved ability to recuperate from any injuries. In spirituality it is used to gain control of the mind and then to flood it and the soul with energy to help them attain wisdom and enlightenment.

In China it is estimated that up to 160 million Chinese people practice Qi Gong exercises every day. They can often be seen practicing the movements and meditating in parks first thing in the morning before they go off to work.

There are many thousands of Qi Gong exercises and routines, such as Zhan Zhuang, a group of still postures used to gather energy; and the Ba Duan Jin, a set of moving exercises which help to stimulate and circulate energy through specific organs and pathways in the body.

Why practice Qi Gong ?

By boosting and increasing energy every single part of the body and mind are enhanced...

1) With more energy it is easier to think clearly and creatively. Mental capabilities such as concentration, memory, sharpness, thought processing and alertness are all improved. With a calmer, clearer and more stable mind, wisdom and awareness will start to flourish.

2) With empowered stronger organs and therefore more steady blood, nutrients, energy and oxygen reaching the mind, the mood too is stabilized and lifted; giving a less stressful, calmer and happier life.

3) With extra power in the organs many weaknesses are brought back to strong activity, thus creating the power to fix and heal existing illnesses and problems.

4) As cells are kept healthy and filled with energy their natural deterioration slows down; Qi Gong is well known in China

for slowing down aging and keeping both the body and mind youthful.

5) When the subconscious mind quietens, both the chattering monkey and the ego are naturally reduced; the soul then begins to fill the empty space that has been created and take its true position as commander of the human vessel.

In general, Qi Gong simply makes life easier and a whole lot more enjoyable and worth living.

In relation to cancer Qi Gong can be particularly useful in these other ways too ...

1) It's great for boosting immunity as it helps to establish a reservoir of extra energy in the body which can feed the immune system if it is under threat from attacking bugs.

2) It will also very importantly help to power the immune system to create more natural killer cells to attack and remove the cancer.

3) It provides more power and energy to keep the body stronger as it goes through harsh Western medical treatments like chemotherapy and radiotherapy. In China it has also been shown to heal the body more quickly after surgery.

4) It will furthermore help to keep the mind and will power stronger to be able to get through emotionally draining Western treatments.

5) It can help to lower inflammation as it helps to release toxins from the lungs and bloodstream during the deep breathing techniques used in its practice.

This helps to keep the pathways in the body cleaner and more open too.

6) Some of the extra energy created and gathered in the body during practice will also be used by the organs and lymph system to clean up and eliminate toxins and open pathways.

This will help both the body to attack and naturally remove the cancer more effectively and also Western treatments to work more efficiently too.

7) Cancer cells cannot survive when they are properly oxygenated. The increase and flooding of the body's cells with oxygen during Qi Gong practice may additionally help in the destruction of cancer cells in the body.

How Qi Gong works ...

Qi Gong charges and generates energy in our bodies through many different ways...

1) For starters there is the breathing technique used while practicing; it is of course complete breathing, using both the lungs and the abdomen to inhale, hold and push oxygen through our systems. Oxygen is energy and as it floods through our bodies and minds it invigorates every living cell.

It additionally allows our bodies to pull extra electrons through the air into them which further encourages and builds a healthy electrical field and charge in our systems.

2) By deep breathing we are also cleansing toxins and carbon from our bloodstream, this allows more energy to gather as less power is required to carry out functioning in an unpolluted less burdened system.

3) With the right posture both energy and nutrients can also move and perform more effectively, thus again saving them from being needlessly used up and squandered. With Qi Gong postures we are talking about opening up the circulatory system, the lymph system, the nervous system and also the energetic system, throughout the body and particularly along and around the spine.

4) Next up, we generate energy through a slight amount of tension as we hold our Qi Gong stance. This is the right amount of resistance to stimulate, strengthen and move our energy, but is not enough to start using it up and weakening it.

When we do normal exercises we start to feel hot as we increase our energy levels to perform whatever workout or activity we are attempting. Unfortunately, by the time the exercise is finished we have pushed ourselves too far and have used up all the energy that was created. This usually ends up leaving us feeling tired and depleted.

However every time we have a Qi Gong session we will generate a smaller amount of energy, but in this case we will keep it all; and slowly over repeated practice it starts to accumulate in our bodies. After a time we have built up enough energy to easily perform all our daily requirements and then also to have a back-up reserve of energy; which can be used anytime we are threatened by external events, such as accidents, attacks by virus and bacteria, stressful situations, or even a particularly hard day's work and so on.

5) In yet another way Qi Gong generates extra energy by controlling the mind and the emotions more efficiently.

When our minds are quiet, relaxed and at peace, then the chattering monkey of the subconscious consumes far less energy.

Whereas the more anxious and wound up your mind is, the more energy is used up and wasted as uncontrolled thoughts flow back and forth from the subconscious. Particularly damaging are negative emotions which can easily eat up your power and drain you of life; to see this effect just think of how tired and weak you feel after a shock or after an argument.

6) Finally, by removing those negative emotions and using meditations to replace them with positive ones, this will also give you a big energy boost. Think of how brimming with life and energy you are when you feel happy and things are going well for you. Through Qi Gong you can manipulate the mind to induce this state at all times.

How to feel energy...

When performing Qi Gong it is very common to feel Qi. Especially if you have been practicing it for a while and have developed the ability to easily gather energy.

Qi often feels like a tingling warm sensation as it passes through and builds up in certain parts of your body.

There is a very simple exercise you can do to feel energy, it works very quickly for most people who try it...

To do the exercise stand up straight in a warm, well ventilated room, and start to take long, slow, deep breaths (try to take longer inhales than exhales, so it seems like you are taking more oxygen in to you than you are releasing back out).

Then after a couple of minutes bring your hands (with the palms facing each other) close together and start to bring them very slowly in and out (without letting them touch each other). Continue to take long breaths, separating the hands as you breathe in and bringing them towards each other as you breathe out.

After a few minutes of this, most people will start to feel an invisible pressure beginning to build up between their hands. It sometimes feels like the way two magnets with the same magnetic poles being brought together invisibly force each other apart. Inside their hands, there may be feelings of tingling, pulsing, warmth or heat. The air between the hands may feel heavier and denser.

Now take one hand and hold it an inch or two above the other, then continue to breathe deeply and very slowly move your hand up and over your exposed arm. Again most people will feel sensations without it touching the bare skin on their arm. This is the Qi that they are feeling.

How to do Qi Gong...

Qi Gong is not that hard to learn. The best way to pick up the movements and stances is in a class given by a Qi Gong Master; but you can buy and learn it from an instructional book and dvd, or these days there are even websites on the internet detailing lots of Qi Gong moves.

There are many different exercises and styles; each teacher will have their own personal techniques to show you.

My favorites systems are the Ba Duan Jin and Zhan Zhuang, they are two ancient and well known styles. However I have also learnt many other types from several different highly qualified Masters. But don't get too hung up on any particular style, as most systems are not much better than each other. **The most important thing is not to learn this style or that one but to practice diligently whichever style you do learn**. The more time you put in the stronger your Qi energy will become.

Although the movements and posture are important they are only one part of Qi Gong, both the breathing and meditation that goes with them are of equal or perhaps even greater importance. So as long as your movements are reasonably performed then you should achieve good results by focusing on the meditation and the breathing aspects. For me the most important part for a beginner to concentrate on is the breath; make sure you are breathing correctly in the way we discussed in earlier chapters.

General tips for good Qi Gong routines...

1) Qi Gong is normally performed standing but if you are too weak or recovering from illness you can sit or even lie down

and try to hold a posture from that position. You will find it quite easy to do proper breathing when you are lying down.

2) Try to find a quiet area where you won't be disturbed to do your practice. Outside in fresh clean air is ideal; but it is ok to practice indoors too, however if you do then open a window and let some air circulate in and around you. If the air is cold be sure to wrap up well and keep yourself warm. Loosen your belt and try to wear loose unrestrictive clothing if you can.

3) As you will usually be standing in each Qi Gong pose for a set period of time, it is best to get yourself a watch or an alarm with some sort of count-down timer on it. This is much better than having to keep distracting yourself by having to repeatedly check a clock to see when to switch poses and finish up the routine.

4) When you initially start Qi Gong you might find it difficult to keep quiet or you might even be disturbed by the quiet itself. If this is the case you can have music playing softly in the background; but do choose music that has no chorus or anything to sing along too, so the mind can't join in with it. Gentle classical music is often ideal as it distracts and leads the mind rather than allowing it to co-create the music.

5) The best and easiest time to practice Qi Gong is usually first thing in the morning. If you put it off until later in the day you may often find you don't manage to get around to it, and the whole day slips by without your Qi Gong session. As Qi Gong gradually and slowly accumulates the energy in the

body, **it is essential to do it nearly every day** to achieve positive productive effects. So getting your practice over and done with first thing in the morning is for most people the best way to keep to a steady routine and achieve this.

6) Remember with your breathing to aim to try and take in and absorb more oxygen than you are releasing during your practice time. The idea is to flood the body, brain and all your cells with as much empowering and healing energy yielding oxygen as you can.

Meditations you can use in your Qi Gong practice...

Here are a few simple meditations that you can use during your Qi Gong routine; they can also be applied to Yoga or any other type of meditation ...

1) Simply relax ...

Breathe in, hold, then exhale and relax your mind and every other part of your body. **Let all stress, worries and cares fade away and be released from your body, mind and soul.**

Take in a deep breath and work from the head down to relax each body part in turn.

Relax your facial muscles, your neck, shoulders, chest, back, abdomen, internal organs, arms, hands, buttocks, hips, thighs, calves and feet.

2) Simply breathe...

Start to take in deep abdominal and complete breaths, feeling the energy being pulled deep down into your lower belly. Do this for at least twelve slow breaths.

Try to make each inhale a little longer and deeper than the last one.

3) The inner smile...

Create a real smile on your face, filling it with warmth, love, peace and happiness. Then imagine that this smile is drifting down the front of your body, melting through the muscles, filling them with joy and affection.

Repeat this again, sending the smile down through the center of the body, spreading warmth and love through the organs. And finally once more let the smile melt down the back of your body.

4) Bathing in the sun...

Bring the conscious thought up into your head and focus it on the area between your eyebrows. Now imagine the area filling with the warming and glowing golden light of the sun. This energy is empowering and refreshing you. Feel it spread throughout your whole body as if you are standing, bathed in the glorious healing rays of heat and light from the sun on a hot summers day. Absorb its energy and power.

5) Filling with power...

Breathe deeply right down to your lower belly, beneath the navel (this is a powerful area in Chinese Medicine which has a major effect to stimulate the body's healing hormones). Fill this area with energy. Concentrate the minds focus to this point (wherever you concentrate your intent on your energy will flow to). Now imagine a glowing ball of vibrant bright shining energy. As you inhale it expands and grows larger, as you exhale you contract and condense this powerful energy. Imagine this ball is full of raw power and electricity and is now providing your kidneys and digestion with great power to help them function better.

After eight breaths start again but this time visualize growing the energy in the center of your chest (this area has a major impact on your heart and emotional well-being). Fill this ball with energy, peace, calmness, compassion and love.

After another eight breaths, finally create a new ball of energy in your mind between the eyebrows (this impacts your mental and spiritual well-being). Fill this area with energy, intelligence, wisdom and understanding.

6) Connecting to the higher source...

In this part of the meditation, connect to your God. Whether that is God, Spirit, Universe or some other form of higher energy and intelligence, then that is entirely up to you. But feel its love and acceptance and feel gratitude for it. Take a few moments to connect and pray deeply for love, happiness and wisdom in your life.

7) Positive affirmations...

Do these towards the end of your meditation routines when your subconscious mind has become quieter and is in a more suggestible and easily influenced state.

Start to implant suggestions into it of who you want to become. Remember to focus on what you want to be rather than on what you want to get rid of, as often the subconscious is prone to try to create whatever you are thinking of, be it in your interests or not. So always focus clearly on and attach good emotions and feelings to what you want to achieve.

You can make up whatever affirmations you choose, just be sure to make them meaningful and productive for your life. You could say things such as "with every breath I take, I am filled with an abundance of peace and love".

If you have cancer then you must not focus on the cancer but instead on getting perfectly well. You could say something like "every day in every good way, I am getting healthier and healthier, every day in every good way, I am getting stronger and stronger".

When you say your affirmations, be sure to attach a good positive upbeat feeling to them. Repeat the most important ones several times over and over in your head.

8) Stillness and quiet...

For the last part of your meditation, you should try to turn the mind completely off or at least minimize it down to as few thoughts as you can.

It is very normal for thoughts and distractions to keep popping up from the subconscious mind. There are many methods used to try to reduce these...

You can become the observer, and just watch the thought as it comes up into the mind and then moves through it and out of it. Don't become involved or interfere with the thought, just observe it.

Another method is to give your thoughts a quick answer, "yes" or "no", or you can use "later" for any complicated thoughts. This tends to be quite effective and should halt the same questions from repeating on you.

You could also engage the conscious mind to focus on just one action. This strengthens the conscious mind and pulls energy and power away from the subconscious. You can focus on your breathing or on a spot in your visual field or even on a candle.

Focusing the mind on breathing is probably the most common and widely used method to quiet the mind during meditation.

Whatever you do, don't try too hard to fight or suppress the thoughts. By doing this you are in fact feeding them and will most likely encourage more of them. Instead be calm, relax, tell your subconscious that it is being turned off and then just flow with whatever happens. Some days are good and quiet, other days are not. But eventually over time (and it may take a long time - even years of practice), **you will eventually find your subconscious quietens and your body, energy, mind and spirit become much stronger in all aspects of health and happiness.**

How much time you spend in Qi Gong is up to you. Most people need to do at least 10 to 15 minutes daily to derive any benefit from it. A good and highly productive routine would be 25 to 40 minutes daily.

If you have cancer I would suggest you do many (3 to 8) mini sessions over the day, which last between 10 to 20 minutes each. If you are feeling weak then just simply lie on your back on a bed or on the floor, close your eyes, breathe deeply and do some positive strengthening meditations.

Qi Gong is working on long term principles of accumulating small amounts of energy over time, eventually leading to a big reserve of it in your body. Positive mental and emotional changes will only occur through repeated efforts of reprogramming in your subconscious. So don't expect overnight results from Qi Gong, Yoga or meditation. Instead be prepared for long term effort leading gradually to much higher standards of well-being and health in all aspects of your life.

Personally I have found Qi Gong to be one of the most rewarding and beneficial activities I have ever done. Initially it does take time and effort from you, but long term it will reward your small daily investment with a magnificent return.

Section 8 – Western Medical Treatments

Chapter 39

Steps to Follow to Help with Surgery, Chemo And Radiotherapies...

Steps to Follow to Help With Surgery ...

Surgery is often used as a procedure to try to cut out and fully remove the cancer from wherever it is located in the body.

There are several problems it can cause –

(1) Possible risk of death during the operation itself.

(2) Damage to organs and other vital parts of the body which may cause long term physical problems.

(3) Metastasis, where cancerous cells leak during the surgery into the bloodstream and from there lodge in other areas of the body causing new cancerous growths to sprout from them.

(4) Fear, anxiety and stress; which can all have very detrimental effects on the mind and body.

(5) If the patient is left in a very weak state then they are much more vulnerable and susceptible to picking up serious infections in the hospital or other areas.

Guidelines to avoid and reduce the risk of the above …

(1) Acupuncture can be very helpful here. It is particularly useful for relieving anxiety, fear and stress to calm the mind. And at recovering feeling, activity and strength back into any areas which have been damaged during surgery. It can also be very effectively utilized to deal with any issues of pain in any area.

(2) Chinese Herbs are excellent at strengthening the body before the surgery, promoting healing after the operation, preventing infections, calming and steadying the mind, and should also be of great help with preventing metastasis from occurring.

(3) Foods like green tea and bitter tasting fruits will be of some help in expelling rogue cancerous cells if they have been released into the bloodstream during surgery; so they should be taken in slightly extra amounts before, during and after it.

(4) Breathing and meditation will strengthen the energy in the internal system (helping all its aspects work more effectively) and will also calm the mind. If you feel weak and you do not wish to stand then they will still be very effective if they are carried out from a lying position. They are also very practical and easy to do from a hospital bed to help you recover your strength and heal more quickly.

(5) Any time you get cold you are depleting your energy; your energy would already be very weak from having to deal with the damage created by the surgery, so it is very

important to preserve your vital healing Qi by staying as warm as you can in the hospital and afterwards at home as well. If you feel cold at all then request that the heat is turned up or that you get more blankets for your bed.

(6) Our bodies are strongest at repairing themselves while we are sleeping, so it's imperative to get as much rest and sleep as you can after the operation to allow your hormonal system to heal any damage as quickly as possible.

(7) Foods that will generally nourish and build should be consumed after the operation to help encourage healing. Nuts, seeds, eggs, extra virgin olive oil, hummus, cinnamon and mushrooms will all benefit the body's natural healing hormones; whereas white rice, raisins and a little honey will boost energy levels, and mineral filled vegetables like beetroot and spinach will encourage tissue regeneration and healing.

(8) Small amounts of foods like peppermint, garlic and turmeric can be consumed to lower pain after the operation.

(9) Qi Gong will help you recover and heal much more quickly.

Steps to Follow to Help With Chemotherapy ...

Chemotherapy is seen in Chinese Medicine as a very bitter poison; its intention is to poison and kill cancerous cells and to get the body to push them and this bitter chemical poison out of itself.

The problem is this poison also often kills healthy cells along with cancerous ones. By destroying good healthy cells and by stripping away needed nutrients and hormones, it can cause major disruption to both short and long term health. The side effects of many chemo drugs can be horrendous; some of the drugs used have even been linked to causing cellular damage which can lead to new cancers in the future.

Unfortunately these drugs can be so harmful and dangerous that they can often cause the death of the patient before they have successfully removed all the cancer. The two most common ways this occurs is through the weakening of organs which leads to their failure; and through the destruction of the immune system which leaves you defenseless against the common cold or stomach bugs, under these circumstances these simple ailments have the power to cause death.

Western doctors find themselves trapped in a very difficult dilemma: if they do not give enough chemo the cancer may kill the patient, but if they give too much then it can be the chemo (directly or indirectly through weak immunity and infections) that ends the patient's life.

Although you can use Chinese Therapies to help alleviate any long term side effects caused by the chemotherapy, our main aim here is to keep you alive; and as strong and healthy as possible while you are undergoing this arduous treatment. This will make things easier for you as you pass through this very difficult time, but will also help the chemo drugs work more effectively in your body. If you can stay healthy longer then you can tolerate more chemo if needed, giving it a better chance to kill the cancer and a higher chance of survival.

So what can we do to help this treatment ...

(1) Acupuncture can be of particular benefit in reducing and resolving any side-effects during and after chemotherapy.

(2) Chinese Herbs will be of great benefit in keeping you stronger during chemo. **If you can only afford to get one type of Chinese Medicine then I strongly recommend the use of these herbs at this time.** They can be very helpful in providing healthy nutrients for your blood and hormones. And also boosting energy to keep the immune system strong.

(3) Stay as warm as you can at all times. Anytime you get cold you will begin to lose energy and there will be less power to keep your immune system working, this will expose you to threatening and dangerous bugs.

If you feel at all cold, then avoid eating too many cooling foods (vegetables and seaweed) during chemo. When you have them, make sure you add a little extra spice to them to make sure they are digested fully.

If you feel weak and cold then add small amounts of extra stimulants to your diet until your energy recuperates and you feel strong again.

And also eat plenty of mushrooms and cinnamon, they will help to support your immune system and your hormones too.

(4) Continue to gently detox with green tea and bitter fruits during chemo; but keep in mind that you don't need as many stronger detoxing bitter tastes as the chemo is already creating that effect.

(5) Keep your energy levels high and don't overstrain your body and mind; avoid over working, over exercising, over socializing, arguments, confrontations and negative people who will sap your Qi.

(6) Avoid late nights; instead get plenty of rest and extra sleep to keep you stronger.

(7) Practice Qi Gong (or Yoga) often. Do plenty of energy producing abdominal and complete breathing exercises; these will keep you much stronger. Remember to focus on taking more oxygen in than you release out during your sessions.

(8) Do lots of calming meditations to relax and to let go, and lots of health empowering visualizations and positive affirmations to strengthen up.

(9) Quite often I have come across some terrible unscientific advice given by a few Western doctors who suggest that if you have lost weight during chemo then you should eat lots of dairy creams, butter, cheeses and fats; and also sweets, biscuits, burgers and anything high in calories to put the weight back on you. There is not one ounce of science to suggest that this is a healthy or wise thing to do, in fact all science suggests the opposite. You should definitely avoid this bad advice which science suggests may both cause and encourage further growth of your cancer.

Instead if you need to gain weight in a hurry, then take plenty of healthy packets of nuts throughout the day and add in a tub of hummus and a couple of organic eggs too.

Steps to Follow to Help With Radiotherapy ...

Radiotherapy is used to burn up cancer cells. It often produces problems associated with heat such as rashes, thirst and dryness. It can be a very draining treatment which leaves the patient excessively tired.

So what can we do to help this treatment ...

(1) Again we can use Acupuncture here to alleviate any localized problems such as a dry throat.

(2) Chinese Herbs can be used to moisten and build up cooling nourishing nutrients to alleviate symptoms, and to replenish and to rebalance the body.

(3) If you are overheating then during your breathing exercises breathe in and out through your mouth to expel overheated energies. When you breathe through the mouth (instead of the nose) it produces a cooling effect in the lungs. This will also help to flush out dead cancerous cells from the blood stream.

If you are feeling well enough then doing gentle exercises during this time will also help to rid dead cells from the body.

(4) Get plenty of rest and extra sleep to recharge and to help healing take place in the areas affected by the radiotherapy.

(5) Qi Gong, meditations and positive affirmations will of course also be of help here.

(6) Take plenty of cleansing foods to help remove the waste cells from the treatment during this time; such as green tea, peppermint and any bitter tasting fruits and foods.

(7) And finally take in lots of cooling, moistening and nourishing foods during and after the treatment; such as seaweeds, vegetables (excluding peppers and onions), extra virgin olive oil, nuts, seeds and hummus.

Section 9 – Conclusion

Chapter 40

Some Final Words ...

As we have seen, cancer (for the most part) is an entirely modern man-made illness. It has escalated dramatically over the past 100 years, from being a rare disease to being one of the most prominent common ones, which now affects nearly every other person at some stage during their lifetime. It has mainly come about as a result of the increasing use of unnatural chemicals both in our surroundings and in the foods we ingest into our bodies.

We also see that many Western researchers and even the World Health Organization have scientifically concluded that at least 70% of all cancers are preventable through simple changes in diet and lifestyle.

But rather than shouting this life saving fact from the roof tops, the cancer industry instead continues to masquerade itself in pushing treatments that make it billions and billions in profits (at the incredible expense of human dignity, suffering and life).

Let alone do they ignore the unquestionable, inexpensive and effective natural treatments that their own Western scientists and researchers have found to be useful over and over again, but these corporations will also often try to attack any other form of medicine they see as competition. They will do anything they can to undermine powerful systems like Chinese Medicine which millions and millions of people successfully use every single day in Asia and throughout many other parts of the world.

So my simple and honest advice to you is to research the treatments that are on offer from Western Medicine and to take those that seem to be the safest and most useful to you.

However, many of these Western treatments will come at a very high price to your mental, emotional and physical well-being; as they are very harsh and dangerous causing both immediate and long term side-effects.

Anything you can do that helps to **minimize** the use of these treatments will be of great benefit in protecting your present and future health.

So you need to do as much as you possibly can yourself. Use the techniques you have learnt in this book to strengthen your own health and to maximize your body's own healing capabilities.

Every method you have read in this book is entirely safe and will only enhance your body's natural abilities to effectively destroy cancer and to help you recover from it. Use these methods as much as you can, not just to reduce the need for Western treatments but <u>to give you your very best chance at overcoming and surviving cancer</u>.

Create a daily health enhancing routine; incorporate as many methods as you can into it; from diet to sleep, to Qi Gong, to exercise, to sun exposure, to positive thinking and so on. Do as many of them as you possibly can, **every little extra thing you do will make your fight even more powerful in its battle to defeat the cancer.**

Stick to your routine and it will give you results (I have seen all these methods be successful time and time again).

If you have a bad day then don't give up, just forget about it and start afresh once again the next day. If you stick to this, you will see yourself getting stronger and healthier, **you will see yourself winning the fight.**

It takes a while to see good results - they won't happen overnight; but just keep working at them, **all you need to do is to repeat and repeat these ways and then have patience; <u>they will work.</u>**

No-one deserves cancer; it is an unjust and dreadful disease. My heart goes with you in this testing time and I truly wish you the best on this challenging journey.

It is my sincerest hope that there will be a great outcome for you; that you will not just beat cancer but you will live a long and fulfilled life with vibrant health, meaningful wisdom and all the joyous happiness that comes with them.

My best wishes go with you.

~~~~~

Bibliography ...

Management Of Cancer With Chinese Medicine – *Li Peiwen, Donica Publishing.*

Experience In Treating Carcinomas With Traditional Chinese Medicine – *Shi Lanling & Shi Peiquan, Shandong Science And Technology Press.*

Never Fear Cancer Again – *Raymon Francis, Health Communications Inc.*

Anticancer – *Dr. David Servan-Schreiber, Penguin.*

Stop Feeding Your Cancer – *Dr. John Kelly, Pentheum Press.*

Beat Cancer - *Prof. Mustafa Djamgoz & Prof. Jane Plant, Vermillion.*

The Clinical Medicine Guide – *Dr. Stephen Gasgoigne, Jigme Press.*

The Food Revolution – *John Robbins, Conari Press.*

QiGong Miracle Healing From China – *Charles T. McGee & Effie Poy Yew Chow, Medipress.*

Traditional Chinese Medicine Approaches To Cancer - *Henry McGrath, Singing Dragon.*

The Foundations of Chinese Medicine - *Giovanni Maciocia, Churchill Livingstone.*

The Practice of Chinese Medicine - *Giovanni Maciocia, Churchill Livingstone.*

Chinese Medical Qigong Therapy - *Dr. Jerry Alan Johnson, International Institute Medical Qigong.*

Love And Survival - *Dr. Dean Ornish, Vermilion.*

The China Study - *T. Colin Campbell and Thomas M. Campbell II, Benbella.*

The Biology Of Belief - *Bruce H.Lipton, Mountain Of Love / Elite Books.*

The Power Of Your Subconscious Mind - *Dr. Joseph Murphy, Pocket Books.*

A Little About The Author ...

Myles Wray

From a young age, Myles had always had a fascination and strong will for learning useful knowledge and developing better ways of living. By the age of thirteen he began to learn Eastern martial arts and by seventeen he had achieved his first black belt in them. He then proceeded for many years to teach and pass on this expertise he had acquired.

With his desire for knowledge also came a deep longing for more meaning and purpose in his life. By his mid-twenties this search had drawn him to Chinese Medicine; which became the doorway to opening his mind to a completely different, yet truly compelling, insightful and wonderful new way of thinking.

Since then he has lived, breathed, meditated and immersed himself in Eastern Medicines and their philosophies.

He has studied with great teachers and qualified in all four main branches of Traditional Chinese Medicine; spending over eleven years studying acupuncture, Tuina, Chinese Herbal Medicine and the supreme art of Medical Qi Gong.

He has witnessed through his own clinical practice the first-hand experience of the power and effectiveness of Chinese Medicine; from it being able to cure illnesses that Western Medicine had failed to heal; to incredible life changes in patients as they became empowered from applying Eastern philosophies and methods of thinking to their lives.

He is an avid reader of Chinese, Indian and Western philosophy, religion and medicine. And has passionately applied many of the profound understandings he has gathered from the great masters of the past and present to his own personal life. He believes this wisdom has provided him with priceless support and guidance throughout his own continuing journey on this earth.

He has now reached a stage where he wishes to share this great knowledge he has learnt with others in the world. He is accomplishing this through his writing.

He also continues to work in his clinical practice, where he helps and teaches others how to heal themselves and bring more peace, health, wisdom, joy and fulfilment to their lives.

~~~~

www.myleswray.com

~~~~

If you have found this book to be useful then please spread the word and let as many others know about it as possible.

- Thank you.

Lightning Source UK Ltd.
Milton Keynes UK
UKOW06f2345260815

257570UK00002B/22/P